T0314039

Cross-sectional Atlas of the Brain

Cross-sectional Atlas of the Brain

Peter Ratiu and Ion-Florin Talos

Harvard University Press

Cambridge, Massachusetts

and London, England

2005

Copyright (c) 2006 President and Fellows of Harvard College

All rights reserved
Printed in the United States of America

Library of Congress Cataloging-in-Publication Data

Ratiu, Peter.
Cross-sectional atlas of the brain/Peter Ratiu and Ion-Florin Talos.
p.;cm.
Includes bibliographical references and index.
ISBN 0-674-1023-7
1. Brain—Cross-sectional imaging—Atlases.
I. Talos, Ion-Florin. II. Title.
[DNLM: 1. Brain—anatomy & histology—Atlases.
2. Anatomy, Cross-Sectional—methods—Atlases. WL 17 R236c 2005]
QM455. R38 2005
944'.810222—dc22

Contents

Preface

Thanks to the Visible Human Project of the National Library of Medicine, a complete, high-resolution, virtually artifact-free data set of the brain has become available. The high quality of these 1,481 axial sections has made it possible, for the first time, for images of the same brain to be reformatted and displayed in all three standard orientations without loss of quality. The convenience of viewing the often intricate inner structures of the brain without having to make allowances for individual variation when changing views from the axial to the coronal to the sagittal planes is self-evident.

While taking advantage of these features, the authors have knowingly eliminated other components commonly encountered in brain atlases. The aim was to provide a comprehensive, accurate, and handy reference to the cross-sectional gross anatomy of the brain, while allowing useful excursions into the adjacent regions of the head, so that neurosurgeons, radiologists, neurologists, and neuroscientists—and also medical students, who have no little trouble mastering this arcane discipline—would be able to use it with profit.

Although electronic images and interactive means of navigating them are becoming increasingly necessary (given, among other things, the sheer number of images), it is reassuring that one can still see the brain as a whole by means of a limited number of cross sections. The reader's thumb remains a time-proven navigational tool. Every effort was made to keep the format small in the hope that this work will find its place next to computers in reading rooms, on the workbenches in laboratories, and crammed in the backpacks of medical students. If this will be the case, the authors will need not justify having added yet another title to the already abundant literature on the anatomy of the brain.

Material and Methods

All photographs and radiological images presented in this atlas originate from the same anatomic specimen, selected through the body donation program of the University Medical Centre of Utrecht, The Netherlands. The donation came from a Caucasian male sixty-six years of age, without known pathology of the head and neck region.

1. Specimen preparation and processing

The entire blood volume was evacuated through the femoral vein; the body was perfused with a solution of 4% formalin until clear fluid came out. The specimen was frozen to $-20°$ Celsius and the region of interest was trimmed to a block of $230 \times 250 \times 150$ mm. The specimen was then thawed and rinsed well under running water to remove fixation fluids and other extractable materials.

The right common carotid artery was cannulated and connected to a reservoir containing a mixture with the following composition: 20 units of volume of Araldite-F with 7.5 Microlith-T, 60 units of volume of Dilutioner DY 026 SP, and 45 units of volume of Hardener HY 2967. In order to lower the surface tension and thus to allow the solution to fill the smaller vessels, 0.05 ml of liquid soap was added to every 160 ml of mixture. The reservoir was pressurized with air at around 150 mm Hg, and the vascular tree of the trimmed specimen was injected. When the liquid emerged from the left common carotid artery and the vertebral arteries, these vessels were clamped. The procedure was repeated for the venous system through the right internal jugular vein.

The enamel of the teeth was demineralized by applying cotton wool soaked in formic acid around the teeth; the concentration was maintained by applying fresh solution over the cotton wool. The procedure made the sectioning of this hardest material in the body easier and also helped extend the lifespan of the cryotome blades, whose replacement is time consuming.

In order to facilitate registration of the cryosections with the radiological images, a set of fiducial markers were drilled into the skull. A special aluminum alloy that does not produce x-ray scattering was selected; this proved of little profit, for the fiducials tended to fall out during cryosectioning, and the remaining markers were much too coarse to make a significant improvement in registration.

Before cryosectioning, scans were performed with Philips MR and CT scanners: computed axial tomography at 0.5 mm slice thickness and magnetic resonance imaging at 3 mm with spin echo T1 (TE 15 ms, TR 519 ms, flip angle 90°) and dual spin echo T2/intermediate density weighted (proton density weighted) (TE 98 ms, TR 2500 ms, flip angle 90°).

The specimen was first immersed in a 0.5% solution of high-viscosity carboxymethyl-cellulose gel and then in a 1% solution, where it was left to soak for four days before freezing with liquid nitrogen. The specimen was positioned in a mold in a shallow pool of liquid nitrogen ($-196°$ Celsius), kept constant for two hours, after which it was placed into the cryomicrotome for further freezing at $-25°$ Celsius over the next 24 hours.

For cryosectioning, a heavy-duty PMV 450 cryomicrotome (Palmstiernas, Sweden) was used, with a high-quality steel knife (L. K. B. type M-140-04). The tissue was cryoplaned at 21 μm thickness at 3.0 m/min along the axial plane. After every seven excursions—that is, after 147 μm—a digital photograph of the surface of the block was obtained at a resolution of 1,525 × 1,146 or 147 μm/pixel with a digital camera. The entire specimen was captured on 1,481 digital images. The whole image volume has an isometric resolution of 147 μm³/voxel.

In addition to radiological imaging, cryoplaning, and digital photography, another imaging method was applied: 69 slices with a thickness of 50 μm each were harvested from a contiguous slab, affixed on adhesive tape, and stained. A few of these were then scanned and reconstructed as slides at a resolution of 15,000 × 15,000 pixels. For a complete description of the project, see "Visible Human 2.0—The Next Generation," by Peter Ratiu, Berend Hillen, Jack Glaser, and Donald P. Jenkins, in *Medicine Meets Virtual Reality 11—NextMed: Health Horizon,* edited by J. D. Westwood et al. (Amsterdam: IOS Press, 2003, pp. 275–281).

2. Image processing

The resulting block of 1,481 axial images was reformatted and resliced about the sagittal and coronal planes using Matlab (The MathWorks, Inc., Natick, Massachusetts), resulting in 1,528 and 1,146 images, respectively. These and the original axial images are available on the enclosed CD-ROM. The data set at full resolution in the axial plane can be licensed at no cost from the National Library of Medicine.

A total of 93 images (44 axial, 28 coronal, and 21 sagittal) were selected for the atlas. They were chosen on the basis of anatomic relevance and are therefore unevenly spaced.

A diagram at the beginning of each section illustrates the intervals and relative positions of the sections.

The selected images were enhanced and edited for print, without altering their resolution. Their size in print at 250 dpi was determined by typographical considerations. Closeups of one axial, two sagittal, and six coronal images of special interest in the region of the basal ganglia and of the hippocampus are printed in addition to the full sections.

Each section has an identifier (e.g., axial580, coronal675, sagittal200) printed on the page, which corresponds to its number in the complete data set; the respective sections are also marked in the digital version on the CD-ROM, for easy identification.

3. Layout

The outlines en regard were provided in order to avoid crowding the images with labels. Although producing these outlines has cost us considerable effort, they were not primarily meant to clarify certain aspects of the cryosections. Accurate anatomical information should be sought in the cryosections only.

Some structures, mostly blood vessels, were enlarged in the outline, in order to make labeling clearer (e.g., axial-291, #15, callosomarginal artery; sagittal-522, #37, superior medullar vellum). Other structures were not represented in the outlines, such as the delightful insertion of the TMJ articular cartilage on sagittal-130. When it seemed practical, we used the outlines to clarify the accompanying photograph; in other instances we found it preferable to let the ambiguity of the original stand.

Having opted for numbering the anatomical structures, we hope that our readers will find this the lesser of two—or, rather, three—evils. We find them preferable to abbreviations (how intuitive is it to use *olv* to refer to the occipital horn of the lateral ventricle? does it make sense to leave the codes *mxs* and *spalv* unexplained, as is done in a current atlas?) or a thick forest of leader lines (Saint Sebastian is considered by some the patron saint of medical illustrators).

4. Terminology

We hope to appease the purists by having compiled a thorough index, cross-referencing the unorthodox and practical terminology adopted throughout the atlas with the more straight-laced (and arcane) vocabulary of standard reference works. The index was compiled for the most utilitarian purposes.

5. How structures were identified

We like to imagine that eyebrows will be raised when readers encounter minute details that thorough and knowledgeable experts would probably have suspected but could not have identified with certainty on isolated cross sections. Difficult identifications were made possible by means of the multiplanar visualization capabilities of the *3D Slicer*. This research software package was developed at the Surgical Planning Laboratory, Brigham and Women's Hospital, Harvard Medical School, in collaboration with the Artificial Intelligence Laboratory, Massachusetts Institute of Technology, and is available free of charge (www.slicer.org). The tool affords the patient user the ability to cross-reference a large number of images in different planes and to obtain new images by reformatting the data along oblique planes. With its help, one is able to follow any detail (meaningful or, as it sometimes turns out, a mere artifact) in all directions.

For instance, some important anatomic landmarks, such as the central sulcus, can readily be identified on axial sections while being considerably more difficult to identify on coronal or sagittal sections. If the volume of interest can simultaneously be displayed in all three orthogonal planes in the same window, as in the 3D Slicer, then axial images can be used for identifying the central sulcus and for ascertaining its location on the intersecting coronal and sagittal sections (Figure 1). The same principle holds true for the vast majority of the other anatomical structures.

3D Slicer allows for the data to be displayed simultaneously in the same windows, as illustrated in Figures 2, 3, and 4. In the bottom row the same three images are displayed, while the top window shows the sagittal section (Figure 2), sagittal and axial (Figure 3), and all three planes (Figure 4). This makes it convenient to follow the anatomical structures in any and all planes, as needed; the image can also be enlarged and each orientation scrolled through individually.

Although minute structures were scrupulously identified, the authors refrained from labeling those that cannot be seen on the images (such as cranial nerve nuclei). The addition of drawings and diagrams would have been beyond the scope of the atlas.

6. The data

The only anomaly identified in the specimen was a cyst of the thyroglossal duct.

Radiologic imaging was performed after fixation of the tissue and filling of the blood vessels, prior to freezing. Positioning of the specimen in the scanner successfully matched its subsequent positioning in the macrotome. Because the cryosections represent surfaces while the radiologic images represent slabs of tissue averaged and projected onto a surface, however, exact correspondence between them is unattainable in principle. Some magnetic resonance images therefore correspond to several cryosections and were repeated on the respective pages. The same applies to the computed tomography images (acquired at 0.5 mm), although they did not have to be repeated because the printed images are spaced at 1 mm or farther.

Some post-mortem artifacts are also visible in the magnetic resonance imaging, such as gas accumulation in the lateral ventricles and parts of the subarachnoid space, as well as slightly hyperintense areas on T1-weighted MRI, especially in the basal ganglia and mesial temporal regions. Such post-mortem changes in tissue intensity on T1-weighted MRI have already been described by other authors (see J. K. Mai, J. Assheuer, and G. Paxinos, *Atlas of the Human Brain*, 2d ed. [Amsterdam, Boston: Elsevier Academic Press, 2004], pp. 1–2). However, none of these seriously interfere with the anatomical information.

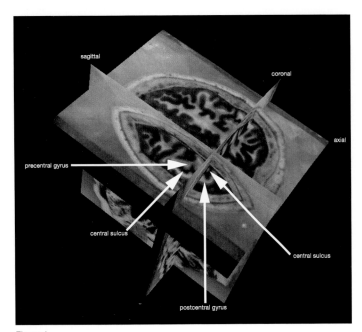

Figure 1.

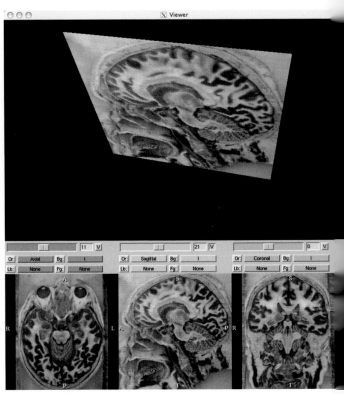

Figure 2.

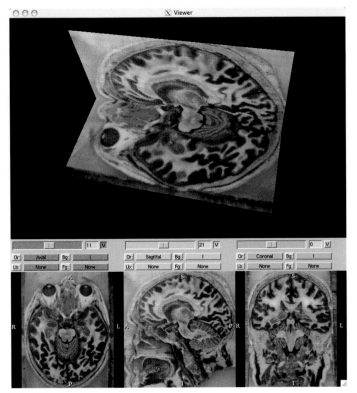

Figure 3.

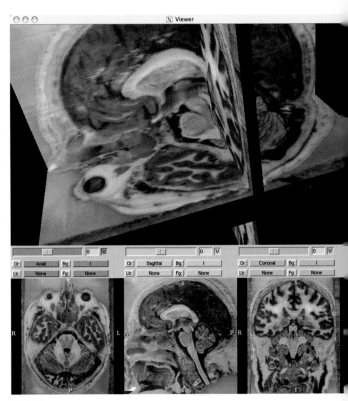

Figure 4.

Acknowledgments

The cryosectioning of the specimen was performed by Berend Hillen, now with the University of Nijmegen, The Netherlands. Steven Haker produced the multiplanar reformatting of the data and Marianna Jakab provided valuable help and suggestions with the preparation of the final version of the plates. Last, and definitely least, the authors thank David Ratiu for helping with the painstaking outline of the skin in all of the printed cryosection images and Paul Talos for his diligence and enduring help with the compilation of the index.

The acquisition of the data was commissioned by the National Library of Medicine, which has made the data available under license. We offer special thanks to Michael Ackerman, the champion of the Visible Human Project since its inception in 1986. The Neuroimage Analysis Center (NAC), with headquarters at the Surgical Planning Laboratory, Brigham and Women's Hospital, Harvard Medical School, supported by the National Center for Research Resources, provided 3D Slicer, the visualization tool that made possible the reliable cross-referencing of the axial, coronal, and sagittal sections; it also provided partial support throughout the project. In return, the authors hope that the NAC's multiple cores and the research communities they serve will benefit from this comprehensive and reliable reference in its future work.

I
Axial Sections

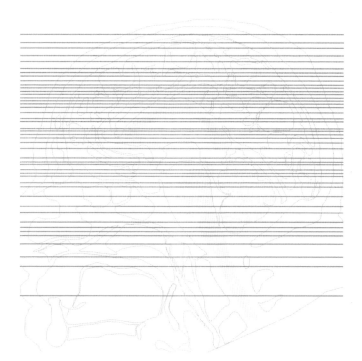

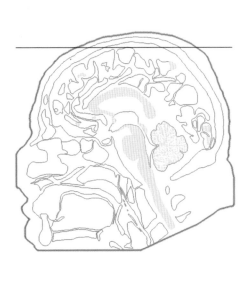
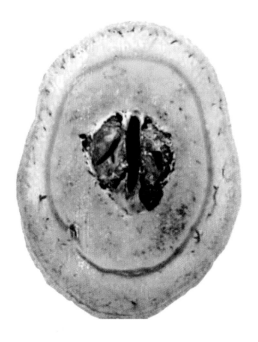
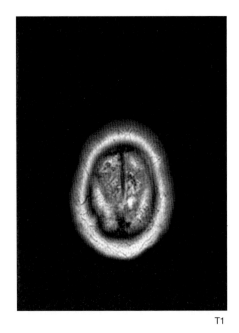
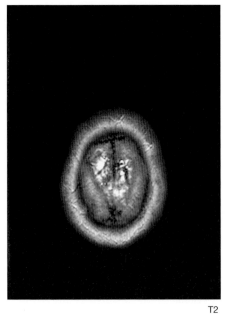

T1

T2

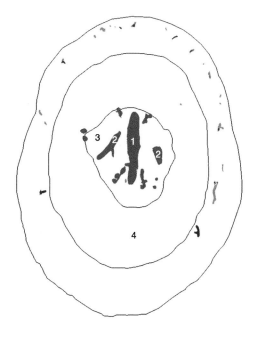

1 – Superior sagittal sinus
2 – Superior cerebral veins
3 – Dura mater
4 – Parietal bone

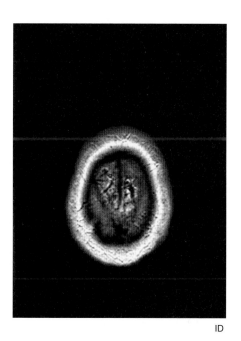

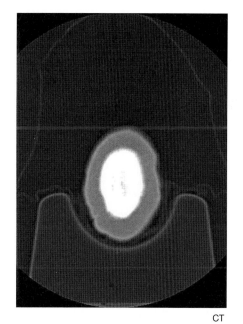

ID

CT

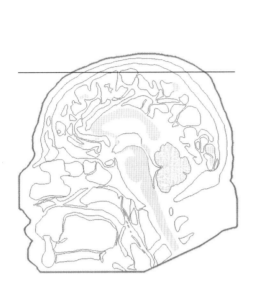

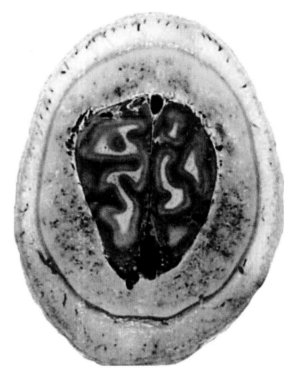

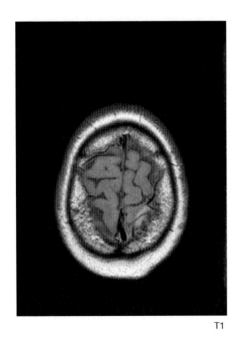

T1

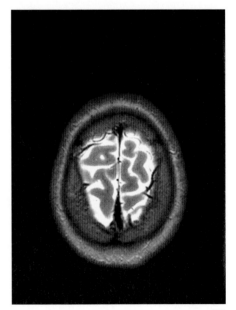

T2

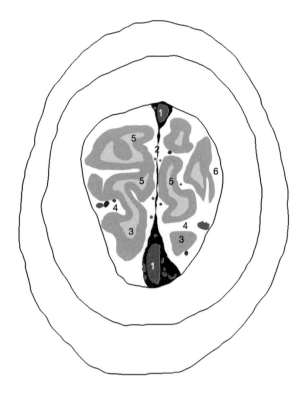

1 – Superior sagittal sinus
2 – Falx cerebri
3 – Precentral gyrus
4 – Precentral sulcus
5 – Superior frontal gyrus
6 – Dura mater

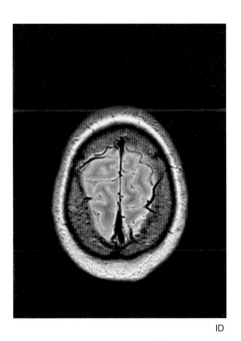

ID

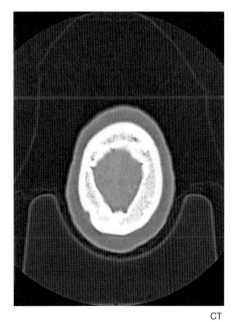

CT

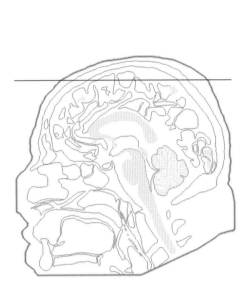

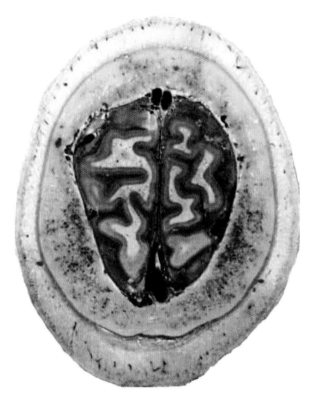

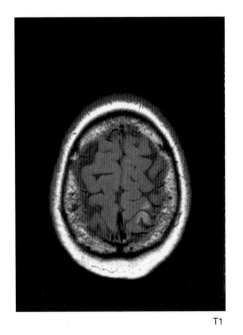

T1

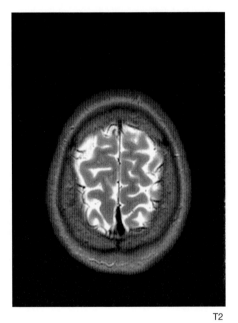

T2

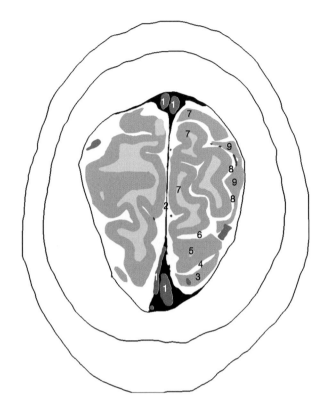

1 – Superior sagittal sinus
2 – Falx cerebri
3 – Postcentral gyrus
4 – Central sulcus
5 – Precentral gyrus
6 – Precentral sulcus
7 – Superior frontal gyrus
8 – Superior frontal sulcus
9 – Middle frontal gyrus

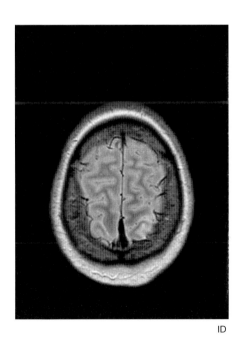

ID

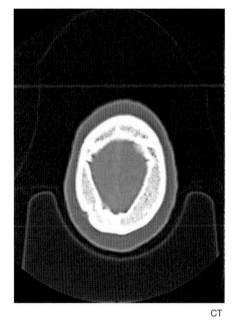

CT

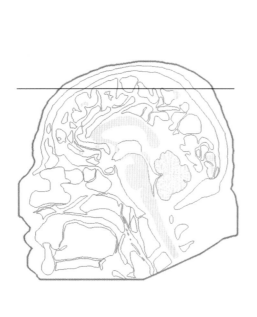

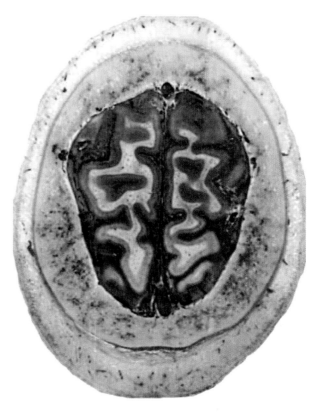

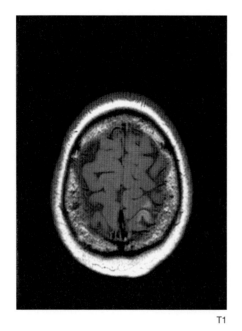

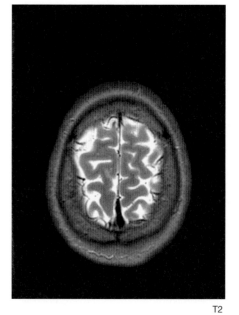

T1

T2

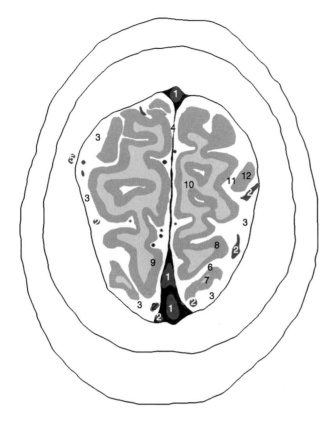

1 – Superior sagittal sinus
2 – Superior cerebral veins
3 – Dura mater
4 – Falx cerebri
5 – Emissary vein
6 – Central sulcus
7 – Postcentral gyrus
8 – Precentral gyrus
9 – Paracentral lobule
10 – Superior frontal gyrus
11 – Superior frontal sulcus
12 – Middle frontal gyrus

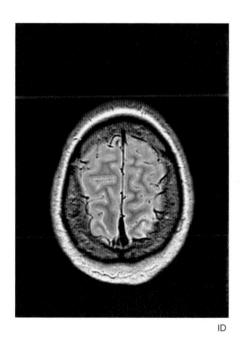

ID

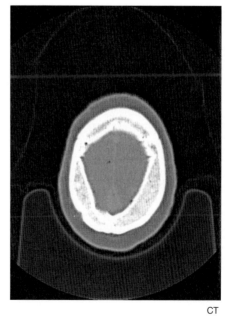

CT

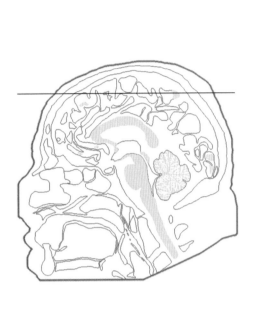

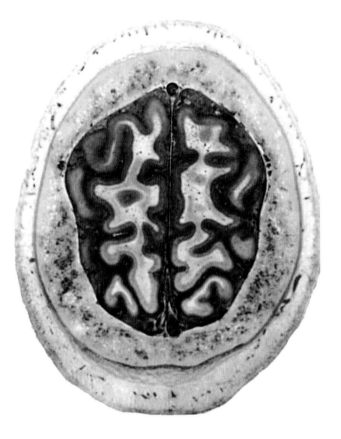

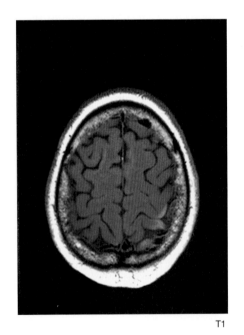

T1

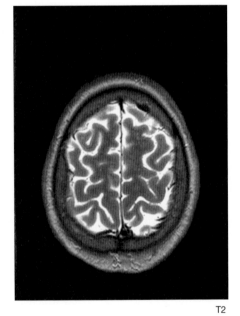

T2

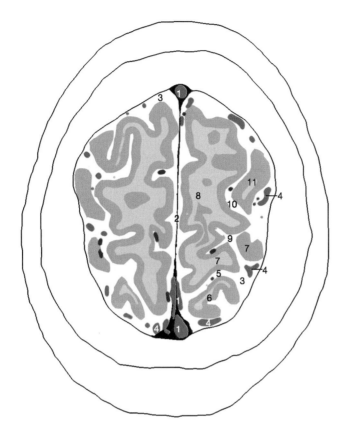

1 – Superior sagittal sinus
2 – Falx cerebri
3 – Dura mater
4 – Superior cerebral veins
5 – Central sulcus
6 – Postcentral gyrus
7 – Precentral gyrus
8 – Superior frontal gyrus
9 – Precentral sulcus
10 – Superior frontal sulcus
11 – Middle frontal gyrus

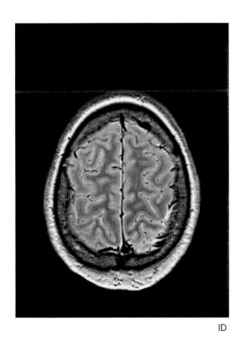

ID

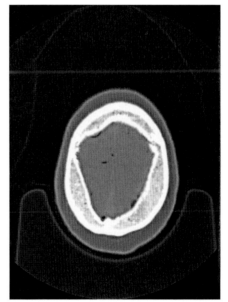

CT

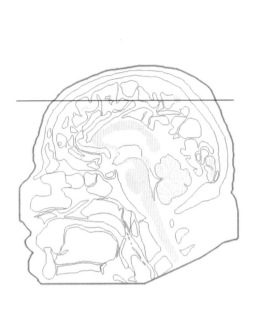

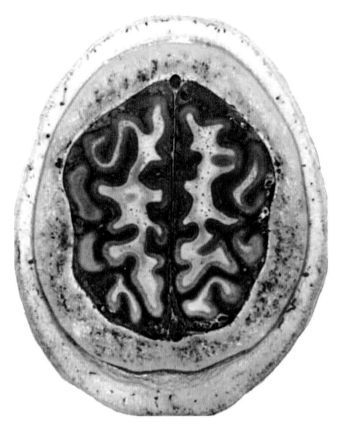

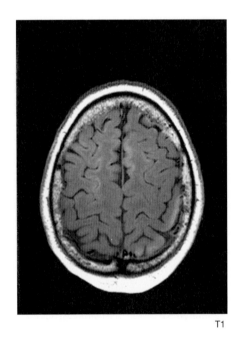

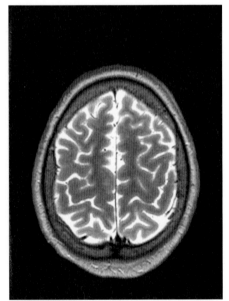

T1

T2

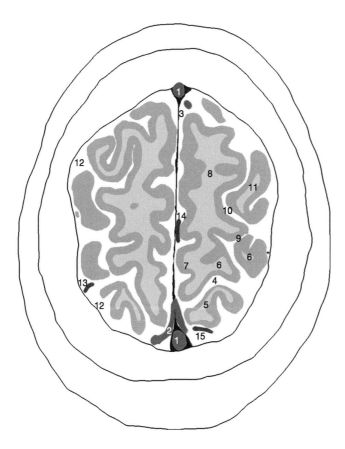

1 – Superior sagittal sinus
2 – Superior cerebral veins
3 – Falx cerebri
4 – Central sulcus
5 – Postcentral gyrus
6 – Precentral gyrus
7 – Paracentral lobule
8 – Superior frontal gyrus
9 – Precentral sulcus
10 – Superior frontal sulcus
11 – Middle frontal gyrus
12 – Dura mater
13 – Artery of the central sulcus
14 – Callosomarginal artery (branch)
15 – Artery of the postcentral sulcus

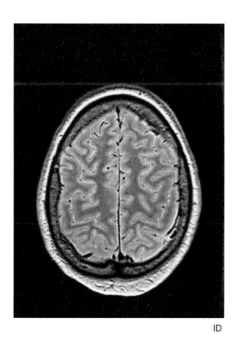

ID

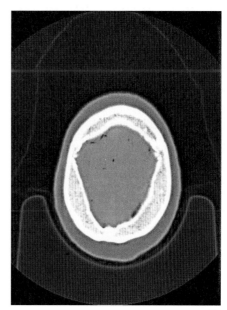

CT

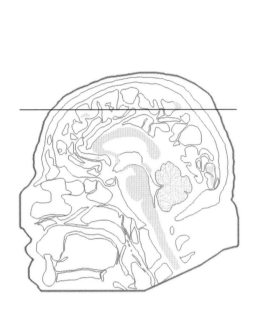

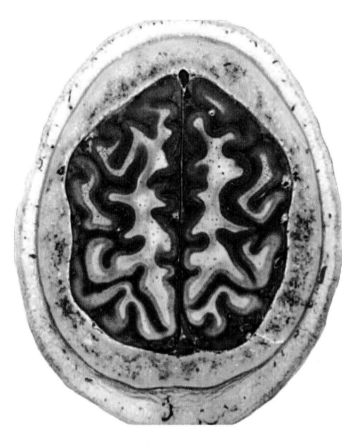

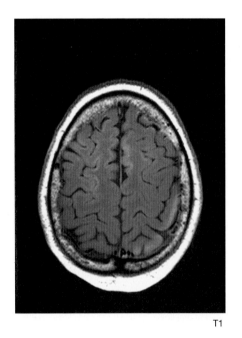

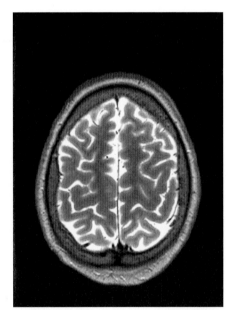

T1

T2

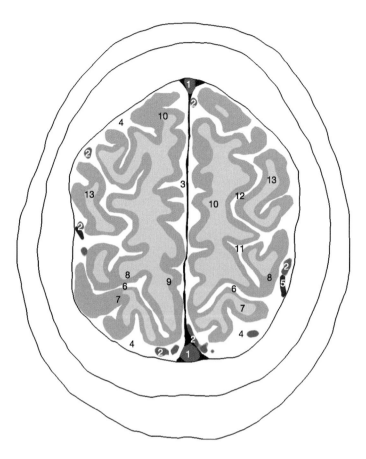

1 – Superior sagittal sinus
2 – Superior cerebral veins
3 – Falx cerebri
4 – Dura mater
5 – Artery of central sulcus
6 – Central sulcus
7 – Postcentral gyrus
8 – Precentral gyrus
9 – Paracentral lobule
10 – Superior frontal gyrus
11 – Precentral sulcus
12 – Superior frontal sulcus
13 – Middle frontal gyrus

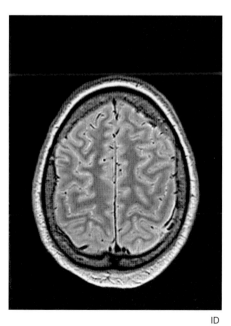

ID

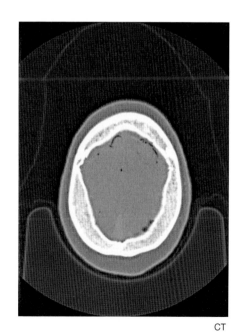

CT

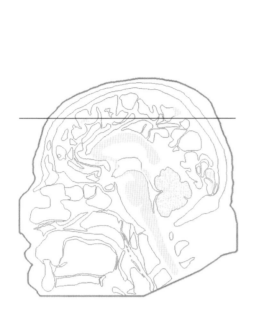

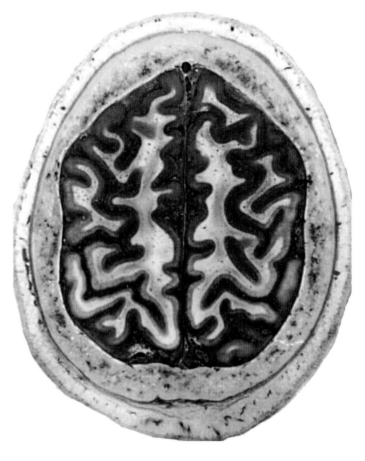

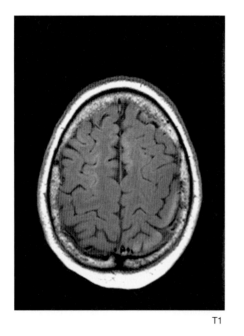

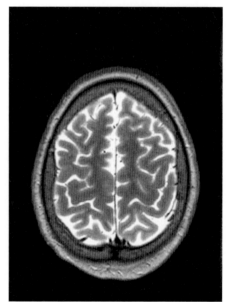

T1

T2

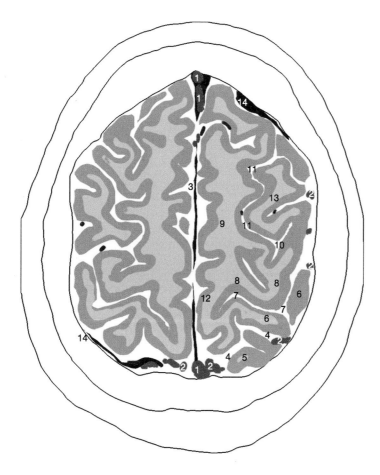

1 – Superior sagittal sinus
2 – Superior cerebral veins
3 – Falx cerebri
4 – Postcentral sulcus
5 – Superior parietal lobule
6 – Postcentral gyrus
7 – Central sulcus
8 – Precentral gyrus
9 – Superior frontal gyrus
10 – Precentral sulcus
11 – Superior frontal sulcus
12 – Paracentral lobule
13 – Middle frontal gyrus
14 – Dura mater

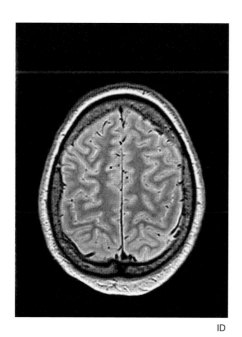

ID

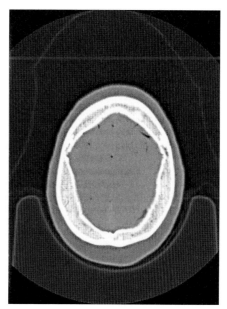

CT

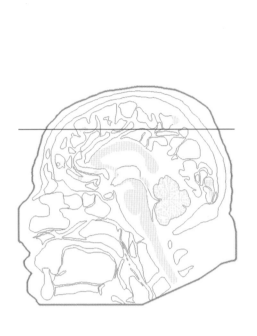

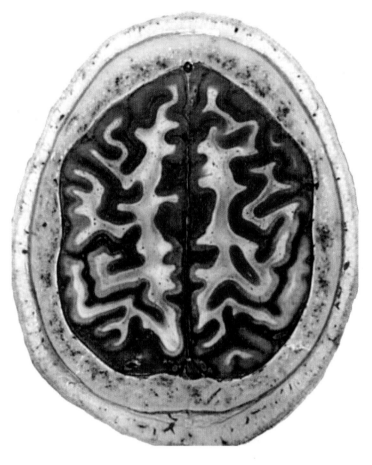

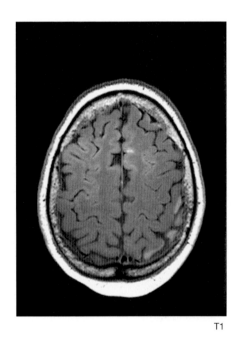

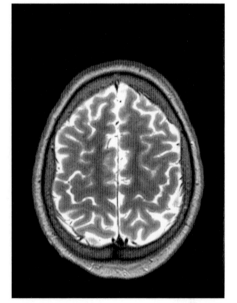

T1

T2

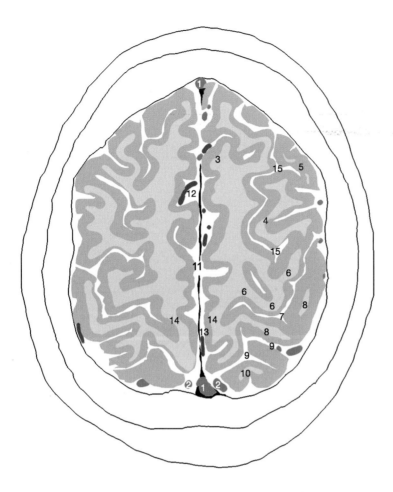

1 – Superior sagittal sinus
2 – Superior cerebral veins
3 – Superior frontal gyrus
4 – Middle frontal gyrus
5 – Inferior frontal gyrus
6 – Precentral gyrus
7 – Central sulcus
8 – Postcentral gyrus
9 – Postcentral sulcus
10 – Superior parietal lobule
11 – Falx cerebri
12 – Branch of callosomarginal artery
       (Ramus frontalis posteromedialis)
13 – Paracentral artery
       (branch of pericallosal artery)
14 – Paracentral lobule
15 – Superior frontal sulcus

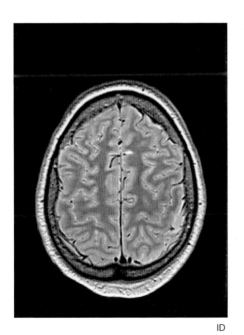

ID

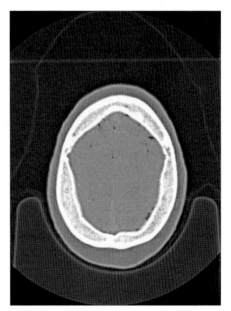

CT

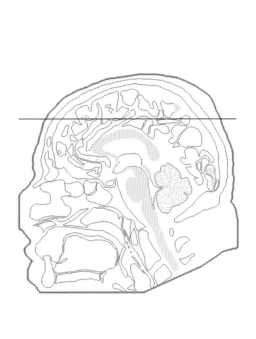

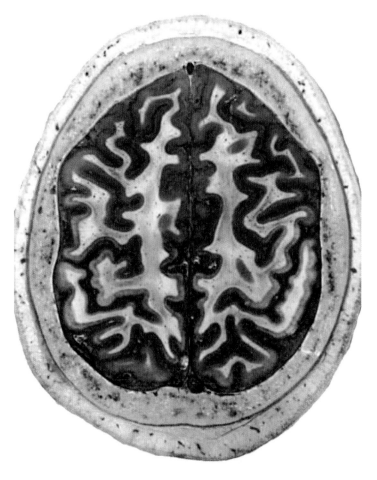

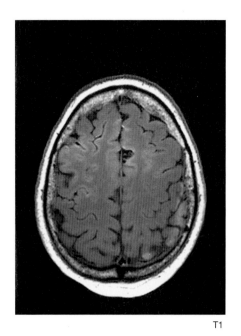

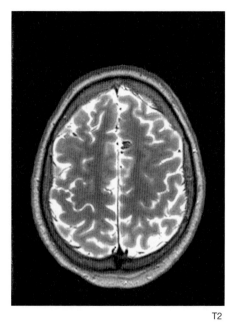

T1

T2

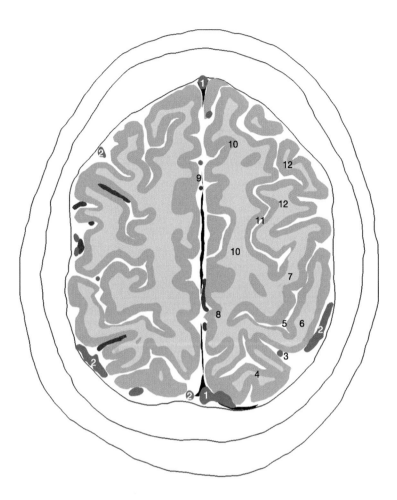

1 – Superior sagittal sinus
2 – Superior cerebral veins
3 – Postcentral sulcus
4 – Superior parietal lobule
5 – Central sulcus
6 – Postcentral gyrus
7 – Precentral gyrus
8 – Paracentral lobule
9 – Falx cerebri
10 – Superior frontal gyrus
11 – Superior frontal sulcus
12 – Middle frontal gyrus

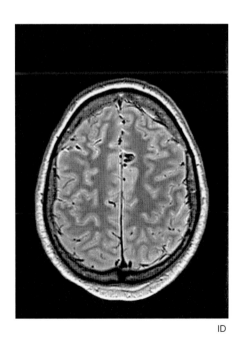

ID

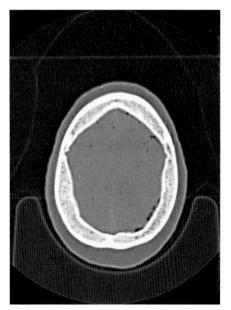

CT

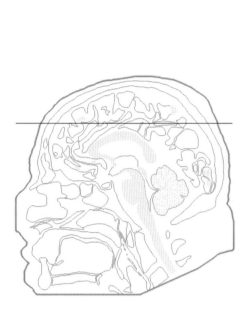

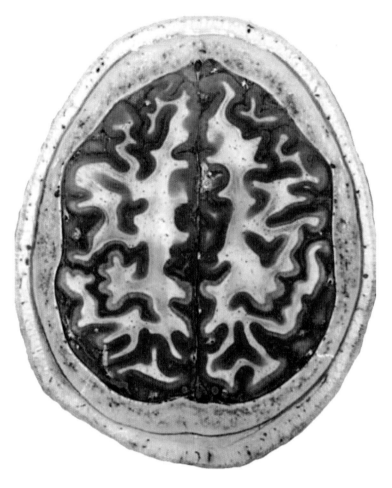

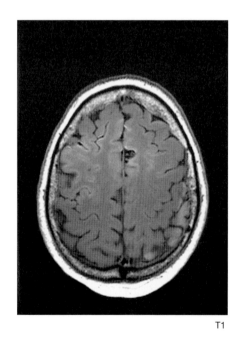

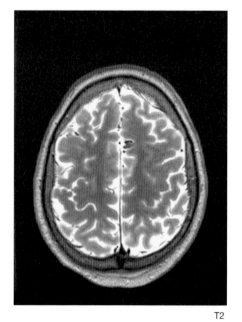

T1

T2

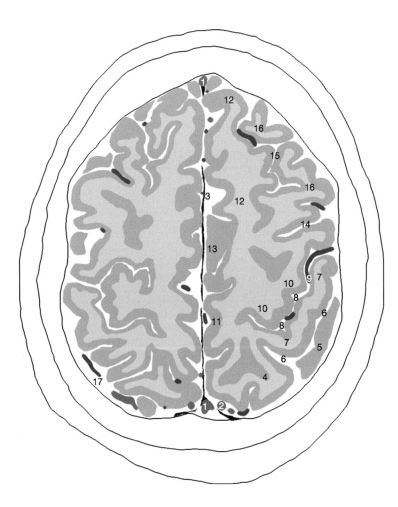

1 – Superior sagittal sinus
2 – Superior cerebral veins
3 – Falx cerebri
4 – Superior parietal lobule
5 – Inferior parietal lobule
6 – Postcentral sulcus
7 – Postcentral gyrus
8 – Central sulcus
9 – Artery of the central sulcus
10 – Precentral gyrus
11 – Paracentral lobule
12 – Superior frontal gyrus
13 – Cingulate gyrus
14 – Precentral sulcus
15 – Superior frontal sulcus
16 – Middle frontal gyrus
17 – Artery of the postcentral sulcus

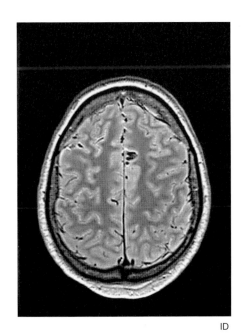

ID

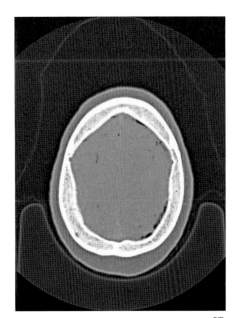

CT

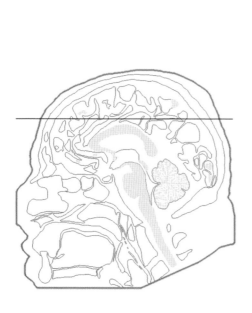

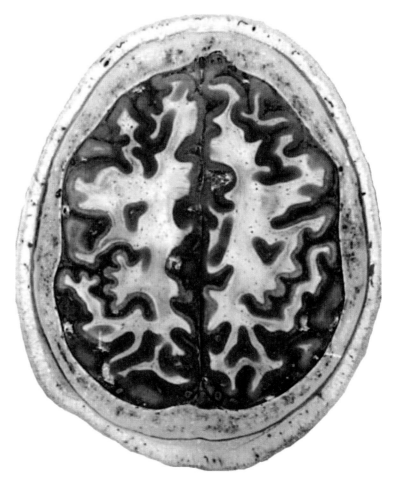

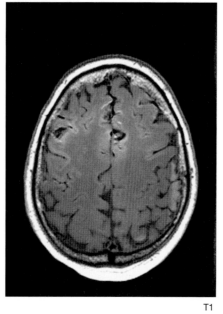

T1

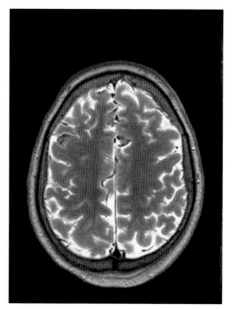

T2

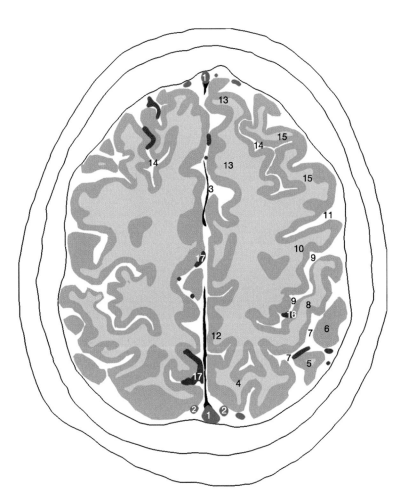

1 – Superior sagittal sinus
2 – Superior cerebral veins
3 – Falx cerebri
4 – Superior parietal lobule
5 – Inferior parietal lobule
6 – Supramarginal gyrus
7 – Postcentral sulcus
8 – Postcentral gyrus
9 – Central sulcus
10 – Precentral gyrus
11 – Precentral sulcus
12 – Paracentral lobule
13 – Superior frontal gyrus
14 – Superior frontal sulcus
15 – Middle frontal gyrus
16 – Artery of the central sulcus
     (branch of middle cerebral artery)
17 – Callosomarginal artery

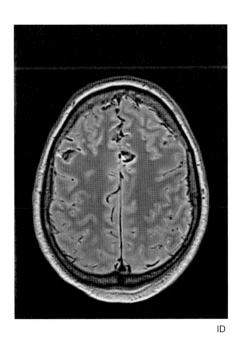

ID

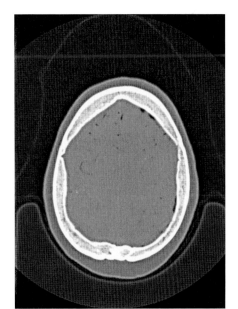

CT

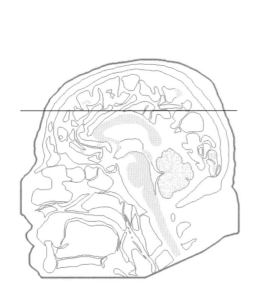

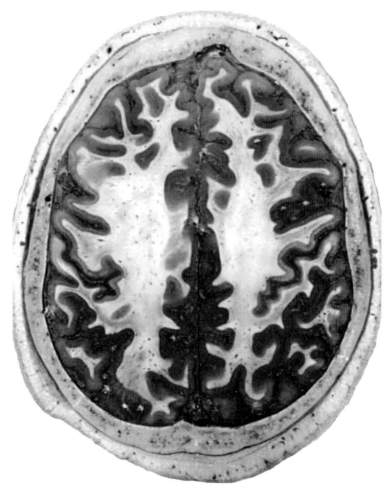

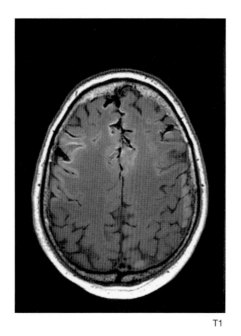

T1

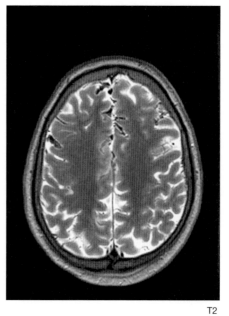

T2

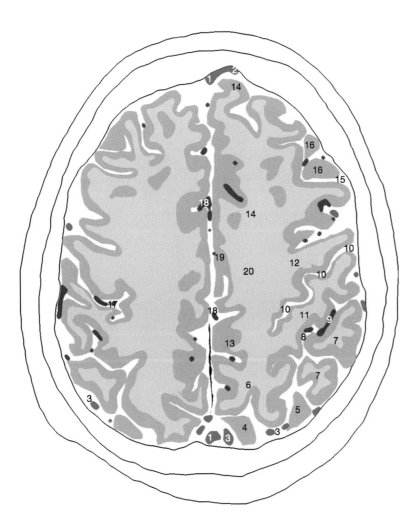

1 – Superior sagittal sinus
2 – Emissary vein
3 – Superior cerebral veins
4 – Precuneus
5 – Inferior parietal lobule
6 – Superior parietal lobule
7 – Supramarginal gyrus
8 – Postcentral sulcus
9 – Artery of the postcentral sulcus
10 – Central sulcus
11 – Postcentral gyrus
12 – Precentral gyrus
13 – Paracentral lobule
14 – Superior frontal gyrus
15 – Superior frontal sulcus
16 – Middle frontal gyrus
17 – Artery of the central sulcus
18 – Branches of callosomarginal artery
19 – Cingulate gyrus
20 – Centrum semiovale

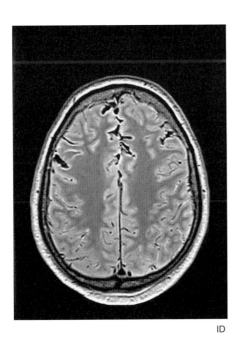

ID

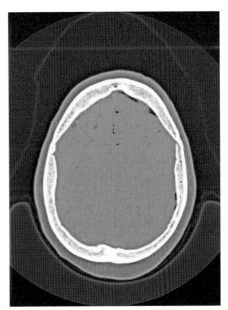

CT

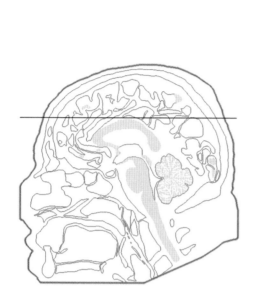

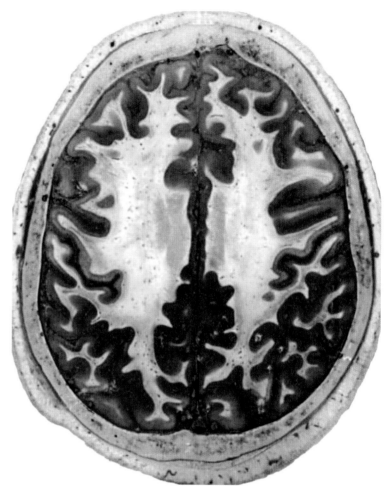

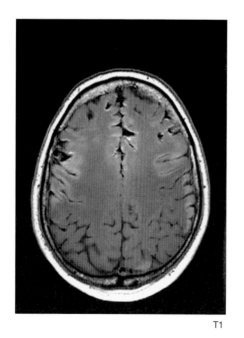

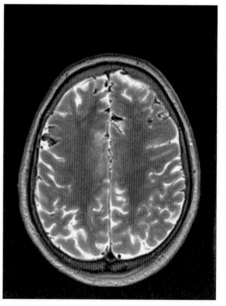

T1

T2

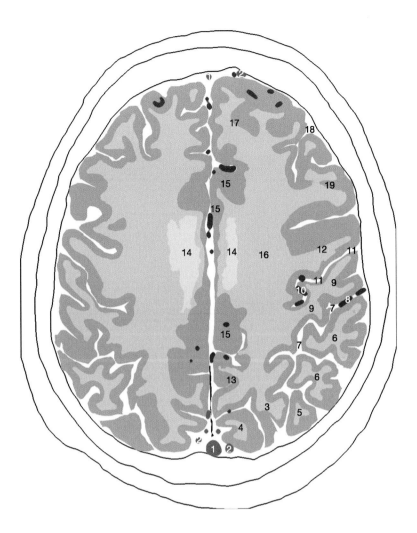

1 – Superior sagittal sinus
2 – Superior cerebral veins
3 – Superior parietal lobule
4 – Precuneus
5 – Inferior parietal lobule
6 – Supramarginal gyrus
7 – Postcentral sulcus
8 – Artery of the postcentral sulcus
    (branch of middle cerebral artery)
9 – Postcentral gyrus
10 – Artery of the central sulcus
    (branch of middle cerebral artery)
11 – Central sulcus
12 – Precentral gyrus
13 – Paracentral lobule
14 – Corpus callosum
15 – Cingulate gyrus
16 – Centrum semiovale
17 – Superior frontal gyrus
18 – Superior frontal sulcus
19 – Middle frontal gyrus

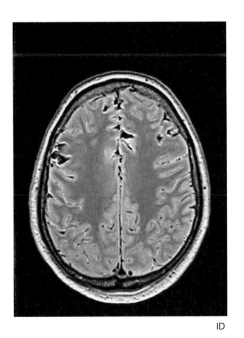

ID

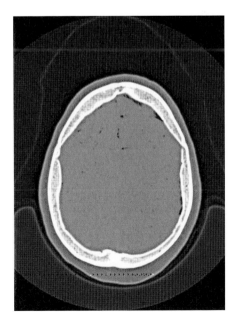

CT

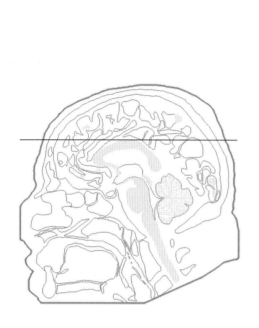

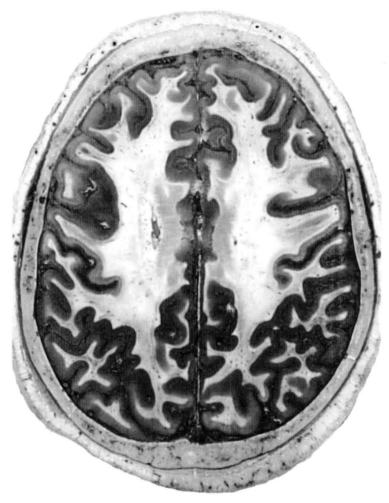

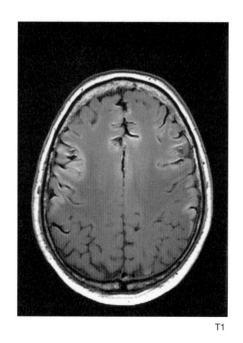

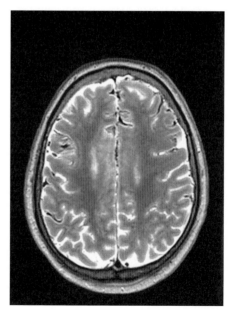

T1

T2

Axial 367

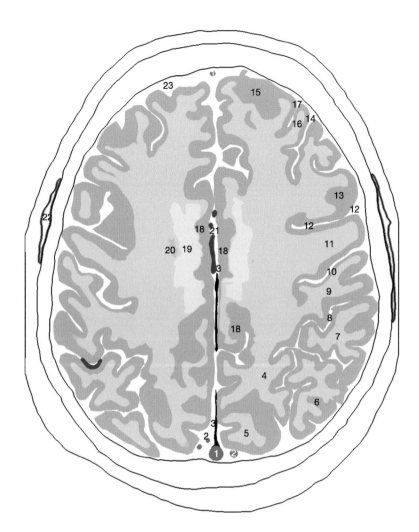

1 – Superior sagittal sinus
2 – Superior cerebral veins
3 – Falx cerebri
4 – Superior parietal lobule
5 – Precuneus
6 – Angular gyrus
7 – Supramarginal gyrus
8 – Postcentral sulcus
9 – Postcentral gyrus
10 – Central sulcus
11 – Precentral gyrus
12 – Precentral sulcus
13 – Inferior frontal gyrus
14 – Inferior frontal sulcus
15 – Superior frontal gyrus
16 – Middle frontal gyrus
17 – Superior frontal sulcus
18 – Cingulate gyrus
19 – Corpus callosum
20 – Lateral ventricle
21 – Pericallosal artery
22 – Temporalis muscle
23 – Dura mater

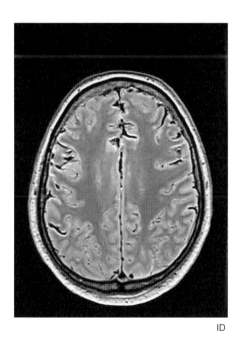

ID

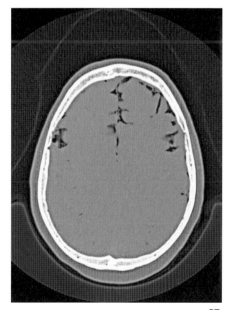

CT

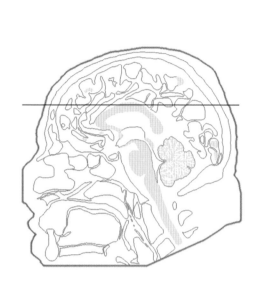

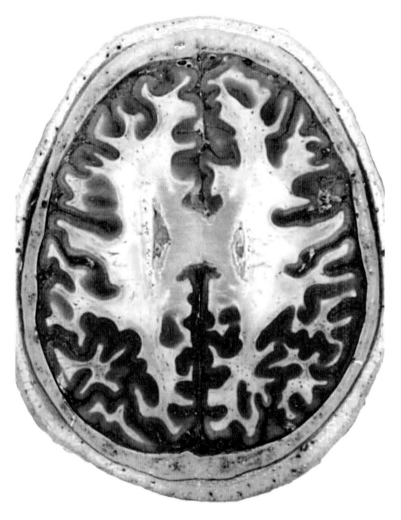

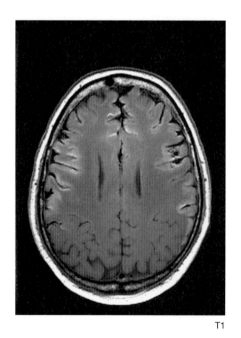

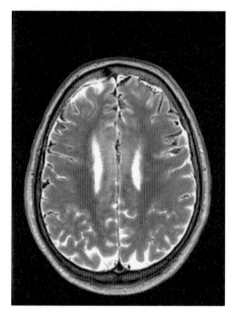

T1

T2

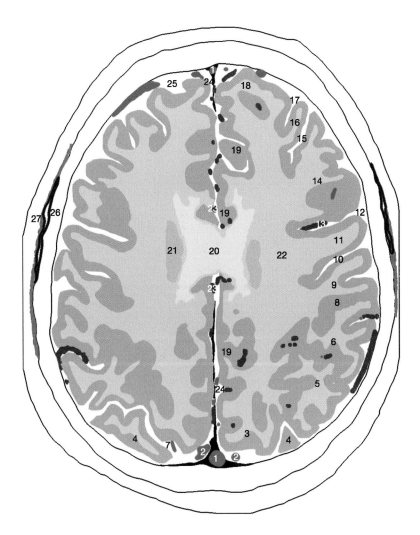

1 – Superior sagittal sinus
2 – Superior cerebral veins
3 – Superior parietal lobule
4 – Precuneus
5 – Angular gyrus
6 – Supramarginal gyrus
7 – Intraparietal sulcus
8 – Postcentral sulcus
9 – Postcentral gyrus
10 – Central sulcus
11 – Precentral gyrus
12 – Precentral sulcus
13 – Artery of the precentral sulcus
      (branch of middle cerebral artery)
14 – Inferior frontal gyrus
15 – Inferior frontal sulcus
16 – Middle frontal gyrus
17 – Superior frontal sulcus
18 – Superior frontal gyrus
19 – Cingulate gyrus
20 – Corpus callosum
21 – Lateral ventricle
22 – Centrum semiovale
23 – Pericallosal artery
24 – Falx cerebri
25 – Dura mater
26 – Temporalis muscle
27 – Temporalis fascia

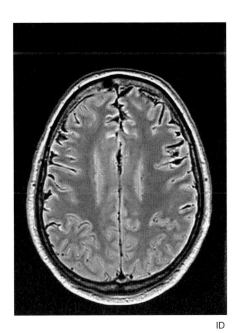

ID

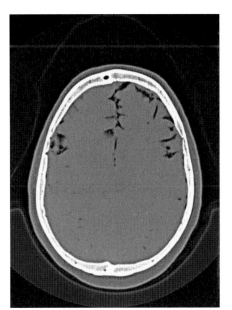

CT

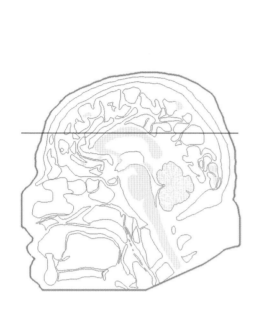

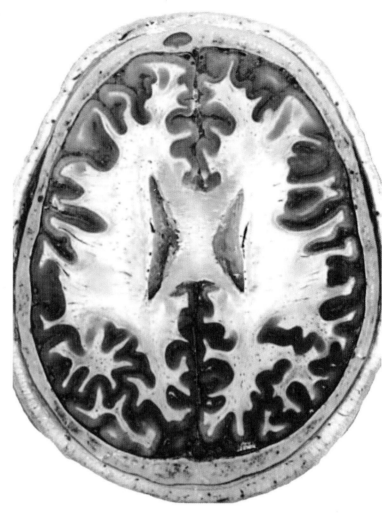

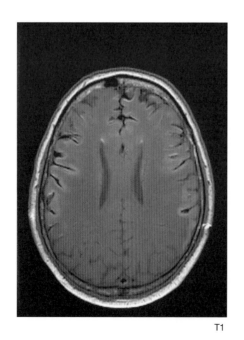

T1

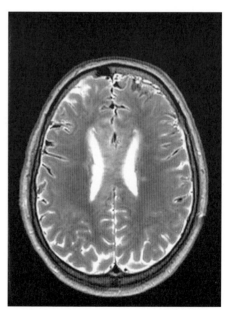

T2

Axial   410

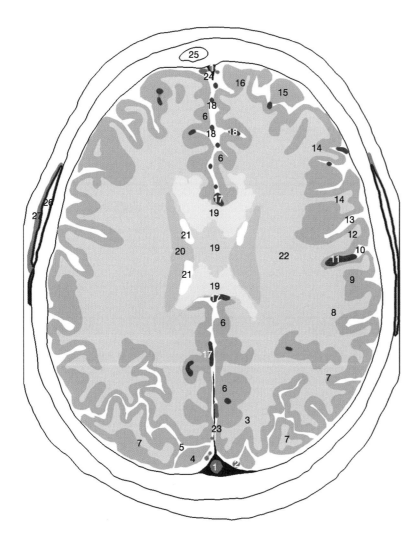

1 – Superior sagittal sinus
2 – Superior cerebral vein
3 – Superior parietal lobule
4 – Precuneus
5 – Intraparietal sulcus
6 – Cingulate gyrus
7 – Angular gyrus
8 – Supramarginal gyrus
9 – Postcentral gyrus
10 – Central sulcus
11 – Artery of the central sulcus
    (branch of middle cerebral artery)
12 – Precentral gyrus
13 – Precentral sulcus
14 – Inferior frontal gyrus
15 – Middle frontal gyrus
16 – Superior frontal gyrus
17 – Pericallosal artery
18 – Callosomarginal artery (branches)
19 – Corpus callosum
20 – Lateral ventricle
21 – Choroid plexus
22 – Centrum semiovale
23 – Falx cerebri
24 – Dura mater
25 – Frontal sinus
26 – Temporalis muscle
27 – Temporalis fascia

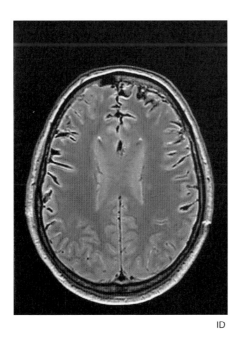

ID

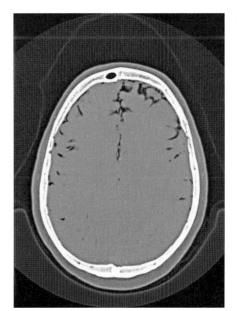

CT

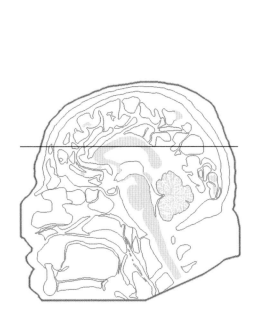

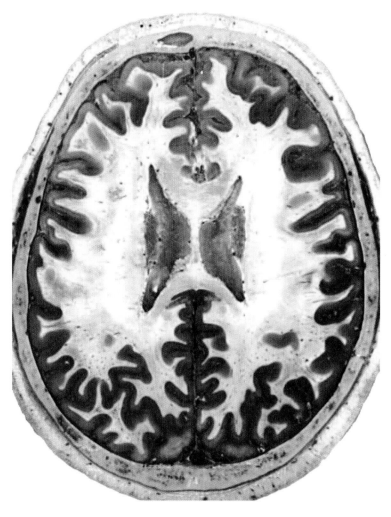

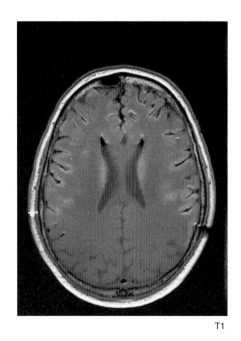

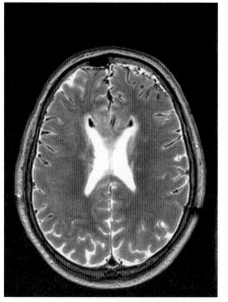

T1

T2

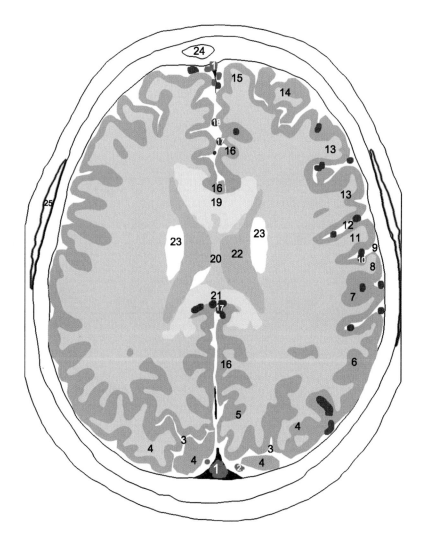

1 – Superior sagittal sinus
2 – Superior cerebral veins
3 – Intraparietal sulcus
4 – Inferior parietal lobule
5 – Superior parietal lobule
6 – Angular gyrus
7 – Supramarginal gyrus
8 – Postcentral gyrus
9 – Central sulcus
10 – Artery of the central sulcus
    (branch of middle cerebral artery)
11 – Precentral gyrus
12 – Preceentral sulcus
13 – Inferior frontal gyrus
14 – Middle frontal gyrus
15 – Superior frontal gyrus
16 – Cingulate gyrus
17 – Pericallosal artery
18 – Callosomarginal artery
19 – Corpus callosum (rostrum)
20 – Corpus callosum (body)
21 – Corpus callosum (splenium)
22 – Lateral ventricle
23 – Caudate nucleus (body)
24 – Frontal sinus
25 – Temporalis muscle and fascia

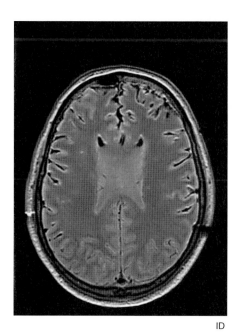

ID

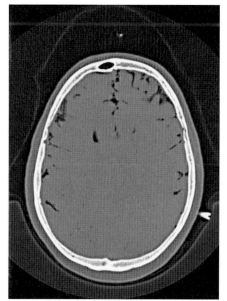

CT

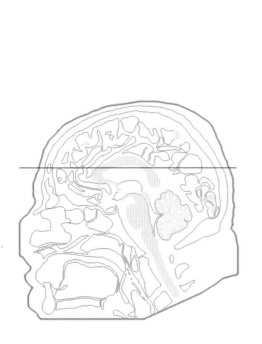

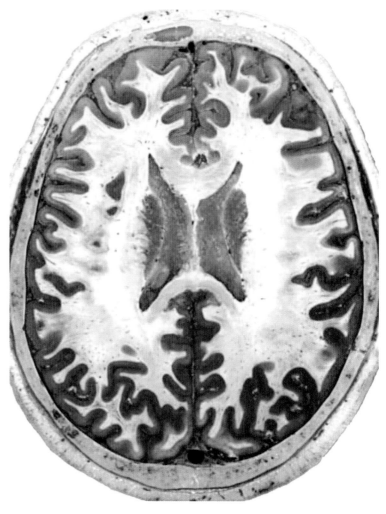

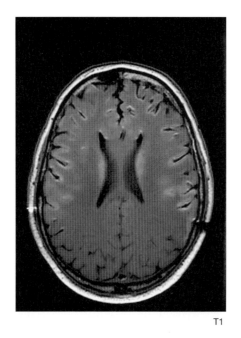

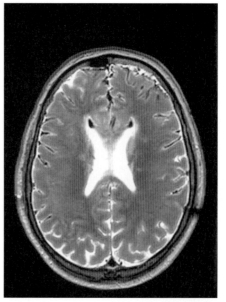

T1

T2

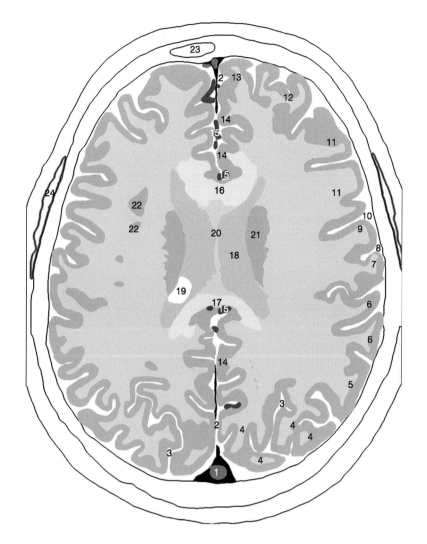

1 – Superior sagittal sinus
2 – Falx cerebri
3 – Intraparietal sulcus
4 – Precuneus
5 – Angular gyrus
6 – Supramarginal gyrus
7 – Postcentral gyrus
8 – Central sulcus
9 – Precentral gyrus
10 – Precentral sulcus
11 – Inferior frontal gyrus
12 – Middle frontal gyrus
13 – Superior frontal gyrus
14 – Cingulate gyrus
15 – Pericallosal artery
16 – Corpus callosum (rostrum)
17 – Corpus callosum (splenium)
18 – Lateral ventricle
19 – Choroid plexus
20 – Pellucid septum
21 – Caudate nucleus (body)
22 – Short insular gyri
23 – Frontal sinus
24 – Temporalis muscle and fascia

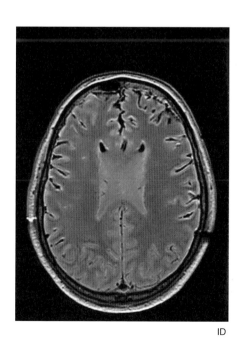

ID

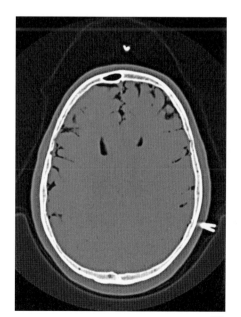

CT

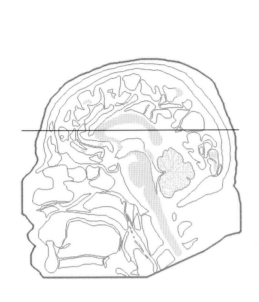

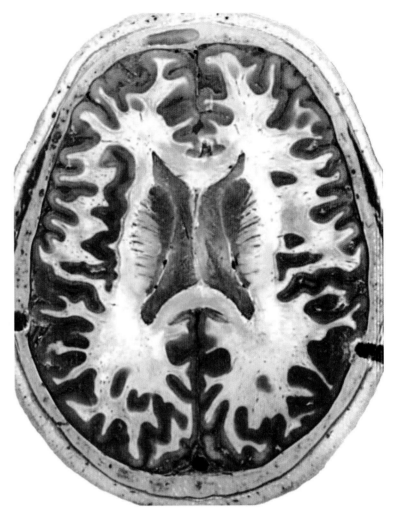

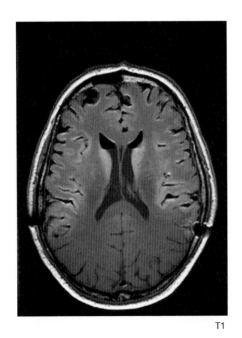

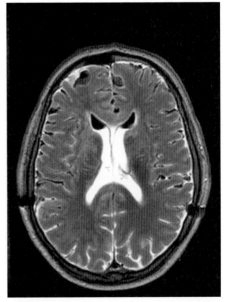

T1

T2

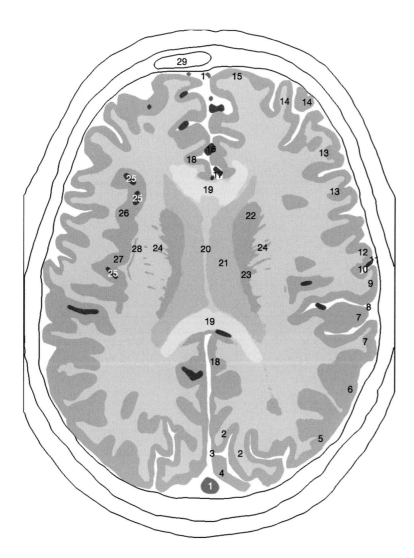

1 – Superior sagittal sinus
2 – Precuneus
3 – Parietooccipital sulcus
4 – Cuneus
5 – Occipital gyri
6 – Angular gyrus
7 – Supramarginal gyrus
8 – Postecental sulcus
9 – Postcentral gyrus
10 – Central sulcus
11 – Artery of the central sulcus
12 – Precentral gyrus
13 – Inferior frontal gyrus (opercular part)
14 – Middle frontal gyrus
15 – Superior frontal gyrus
16 – Callosomarginal artery
17 – Pericallosal artery
18 – Cingulate gyrus
19 – Corpus callosum
20 – Pellucid septum
21 – Lateral ventricle
22 – Head of caudate nucleus
23 – Body of caudate nucleus
24 – Sriatal gray matter bridges
25 – Middle cerebral artery
26 – Short insular gyri
27 – Long insular gyrus
28 – Claustrum
29 – Frontal sinus

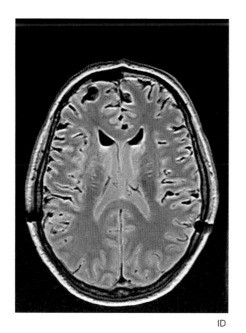

ID

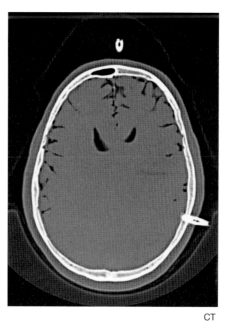

CT

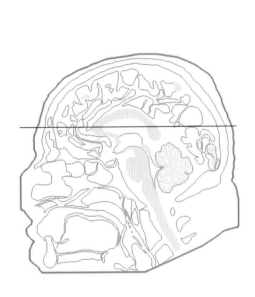

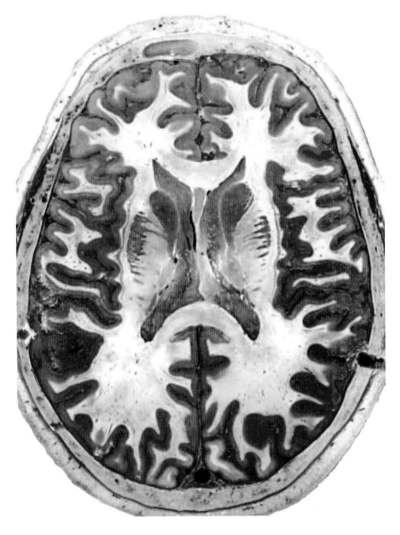

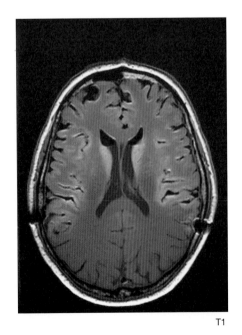

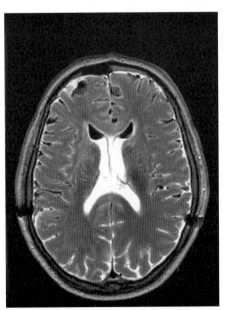

T1

T2

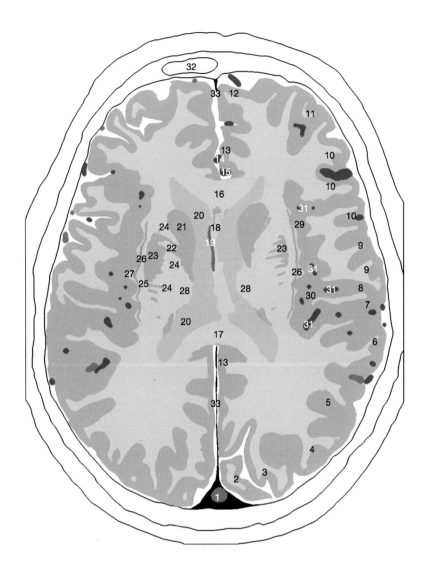

1 – Superior sagittal sinus
2 – Cuneus
3 – Precuneus
4 – Occipital gyri
5 – Angular gyrus
6 – Supramarginal gyrus
7 – Postcentral gyrus
8 – Central sulcus
9 – Precentral gyrus
10 – Inferior frontal gyrus
11 – Middle frontal gyrus
12 – Superior frontal gyrus
13 – Cingulate gyrus
14 – Callosomarginal artery
15 – Pericallosal artery
16 – Corpus callosum (rostrum)
17 – Corpus callosum (splenium)
18 – Pellucid septum with cavum septi pellucidi
19 – Anterior vein of Pellucid septum
20 – Lateral ventricle
21 – Head of the caudate nucleus
22 – Caudato-lenticular gray matter bridges (Pontes grisei caudato-lenticulares)
23 – Putamen
24 – Internal capsule
25 – External capsule
26 – Claustrum
27 – Extreme capsule
28 – Thalamus (lateral dorsal nucleus)
29 – Short insular gyri
30 – Long insular gyrus
31 – Middle cerebral artery (branch)
32 – Frontal sinus
33 – Falx cerebri

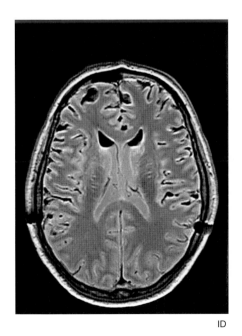

ID

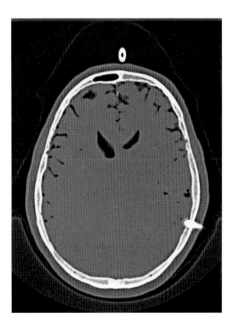

CT

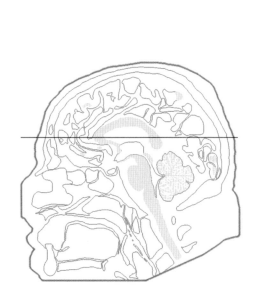

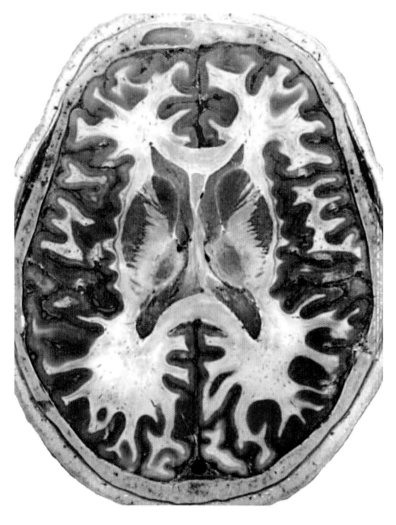

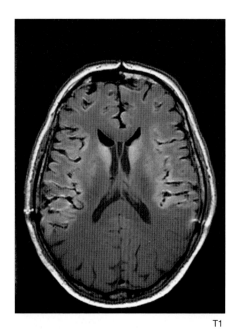

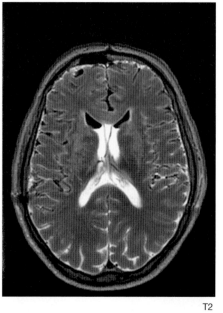

T1

T2

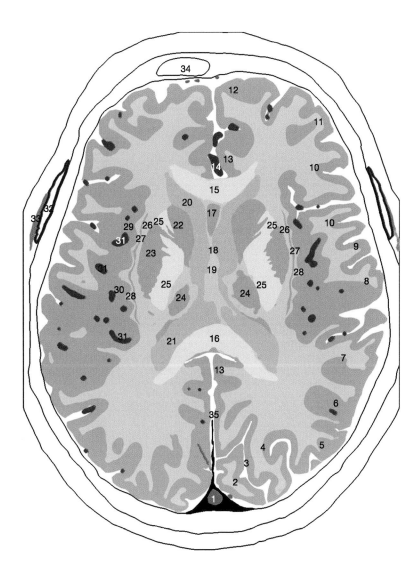

1 – Superior sagittal sinus
2 – Cuneus
3 – Parietooccipital sulcus
4 – Precuneus
5 – Occipital gyri
6 – Middle temporal gyrus
7 – Superior temporal gyrus
8 – Postcentral gyrus
9 – Precentral gyrus
10 – Inferior frontal gyrus
11 – Middle frontal gyrus
12 – Superior frontal gyrus
13 – Cingulate gyrus
14 – Pericallosal artery
15 – Corpus callosum (rostrum)
16 – Corpus callosum (splenium)
17 – Cavum septi pellucidi
18 – Pellucid septum
19 – Fornix body
20 – Lateral ventricle (anterior horn)
21 – Lateral ventricle (posterior horn)
22 – Head of caudate nucleus
23 – Putamen
24 – Thalamus (medial nucleus)
25 – Internal capsule
26 – External capsule
27 – Claustrum
28 – Extreme capsule
29 – Short insular gyri
30 – Long insular gyrus
31 – Middle cerebral artery
32 – Temporalis muscle
33 – Temporalis fascia
34 – Frontal sinus
35 – Falx cerebri

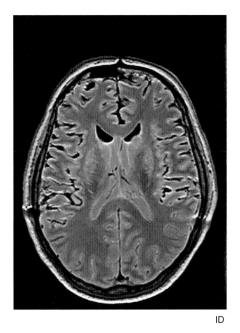

ID

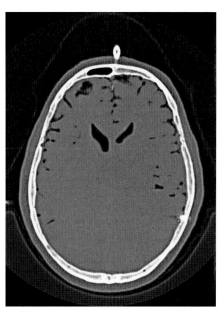

CT

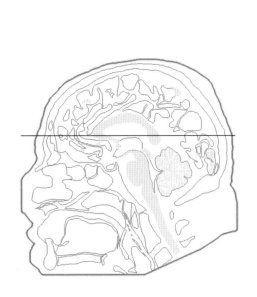

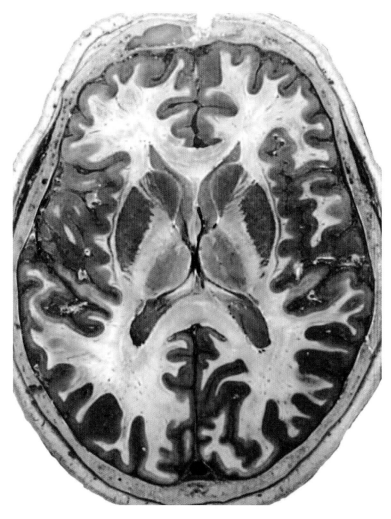

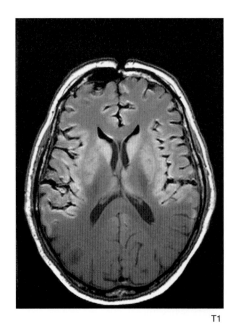

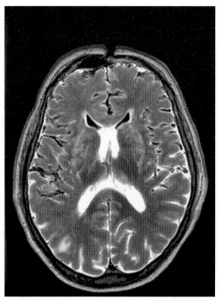

T1

T2

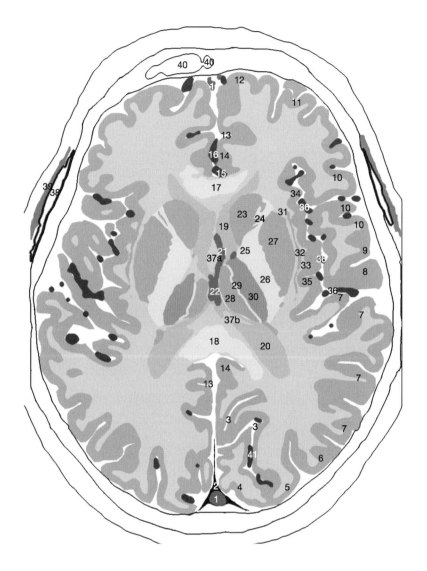

1 – Superior sagittal sinus
2 – Falx cerebri
3 – Calcarine sulcus
4 – Cuneus
5 – Occipital gyri
6 – Middle temporal gyrus
7 – Superior temporal gyrus
8 – Postcentral gyrus
9 – Precentral gyrus
10 – Inferior frontal gyrus
11 – Middle frontal gyrus
12 – Superior frontal gyrus
13 – Cingulate sulcus
14 – Cingulate gyrus
15 – Pericallosal artery
16 – Callosomarginal artery
17 – Corpus callosum (rostrum)
18 – Corpus callosum (splenium)
19 – Lateral ventricle (anterior horn)
20 – Lateral ventricle (posterior horn)
21 – Thalamostriate vein
22 – Internal cerebral veins
23 – Head of caudate nucleus
24 – Internal capsule (anterior limb)
25 – Internal capsule (genu)
26 – Internal capsule (posterior limb)
27 – Putamen
28 – Medial nucleus of thalamus
29 – Internal medullar lamina
     (lamina medullaris interna)
30 – Ventral lateral nucleus of thalamus
31 – External capsule
32 – Claustrum
33 – Extreme capsule
34 – Short insular gyri
35 – Long insular gyrus
36 – Middle cerebral artery (MCA)
37a – Fornix (body)
37b – Fornix (crus)
38 – Temporalis muscle
39 – Temporalis fascia
40 – Frontal sinus
41 – Branch for the calcarine sulcus
     of medial occipital artery
     (PCA branch)

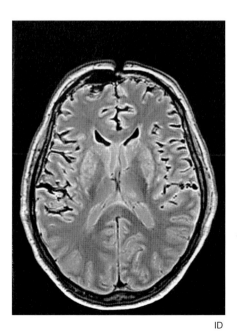

ID

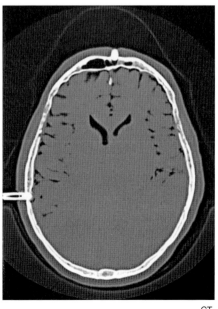

CT

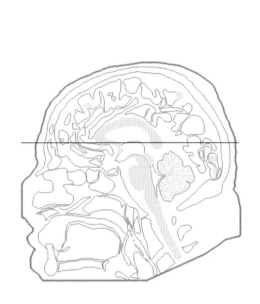

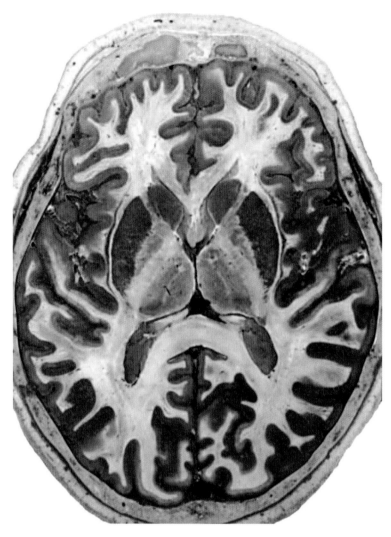

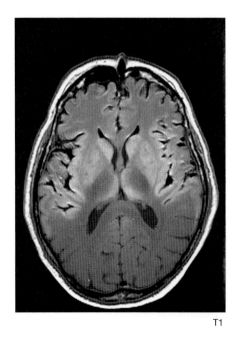

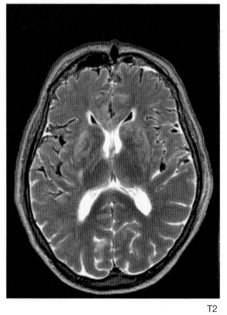

T1

T2

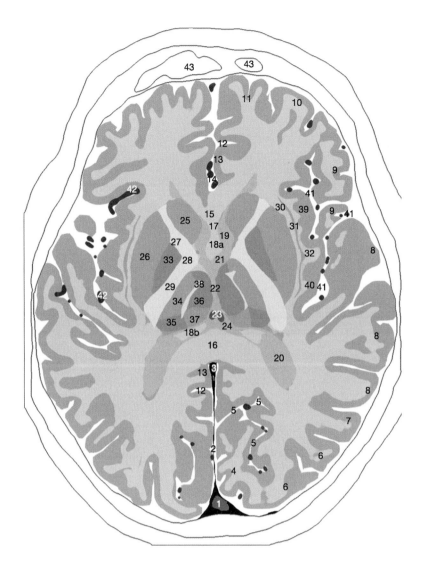

1 – Superior sagittal sinus
2 – Falx cerebri
3 – Inferior sagittal sinus
4 – Cuneus
5 – Calcarine sulcus
6 – Occipital gyri
7 – Middle temporal gyrus
8 – Superior temporal gyrus
9 – Inferior frontal gyrus
10 – Middle frontal gyrus
11 – Superior frontal gyrus
12 – Cingulate sulcus
13 – Cingulate gyrus
14 – Anterior cerebral artery
15 – Corpus callosum (rostrum)
16 – Corpus callosum (splenium)
17 – Pellucid septum
18a – Fornix (body)
18b – Fornix (crus)
19 – Lateral ventricle (anterior horn)
20 – Lateral ventricle (posterior horn)
21 – Interventricular foramen (Monro)
22 – Third ventricle
23 – Internal cerebral veins
24 – Cistern of the transverse fissure
25 – Head of the caudate nucleus
26 – Putamen
27 – Internal capsule (anterior limb)
28 – Internal capsule (genu)
29 – Internal capsule (posterior limb)
30 – External capsule
31 – Claustrum
32 – Extreme capsule
33 – Globus pallidus (external part, GPe)
34 – Ventral anterior nucleus
      of thalamus
35 – Ventral posterolateral nucleus
      of thalamus (VPL)
36 – Medial thalamic nucleus
37 – Ventral posteromedial (VPM)
      nucleus of thalamus
38 – Internal medullar lamina
      (lamina medullaris interna)
39 – Short insular gyri
40 – Long insular gyrus
41 – Lateral sulcus (Sylvius)
42 – Middle cerebral artery
43 – Frontal sinus

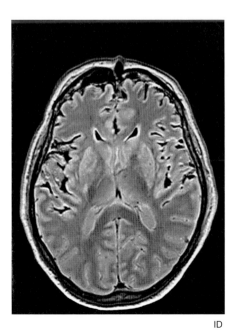

ID

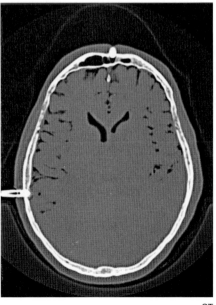

CT

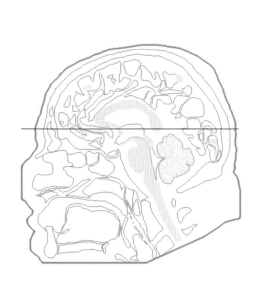

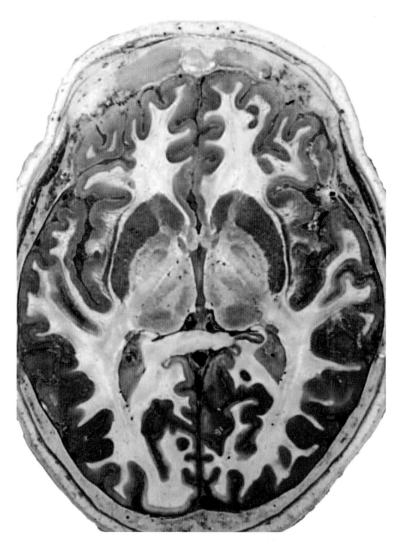

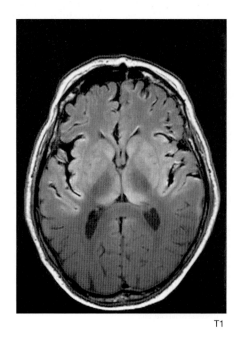

T1

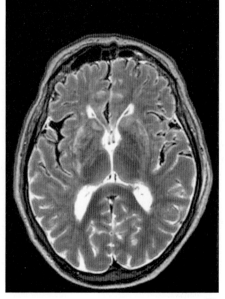

T2

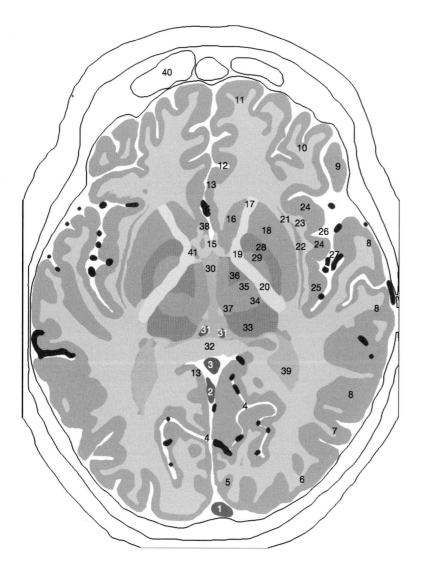

1 – Superior sagittal sinus
2 – Straight sinus (sinus rectus)
3 – Great cerebral vein (Galen)
4 – Calcarine sulcus
5 – Cuneus
6 – Occipital gyri
7 – Middle temporal gyrus
8 – Superior temporal gyrus
9 – Inferior frontal gyrus
10 – Middle frontal gyrus
11 – Superior frontal gyrus
12 – Cingulate sulcus
13 – Cingulate gyrus
14 – Anterior cerebral artery
15 – Fornix columns
16 – Head of caudate nucleus
17 – Internal capsule (anterior limb)
18 – Putamen
19 – Internal capsule (genu)
20 – Internal capsule (posterior limb)
21 – External capsule
22 – Claustrum
23 – Extreme capsule
24 – Short insular gyri
25 – Long insular gyrus
26 – Lateral nucleus (Sylvius)
27 – Middle cerebral artery
28 – Globus pallidus pars externa (GPe)
29 – Globus pallidus pars interna (GPi)
30 – Third ventricle
31 – Internal cerebral veins
32 – Corpus callosum (splenium)
33 – Pulvinar of thalamus
34 – Ventral posterolateral nucleus
       of thalamus (VPL)
35 – Ventral anterior nucleus
       of thalamus
36 – Anterior nucleus of thalamus
37 – Ventral posteromedial nucleus
       of thalamus (VPM)
38 – Paraterminal gyrus
39 – Lateral ventricle (posterior horn)
40 – Frontal sinus
41 – Septal nuclei

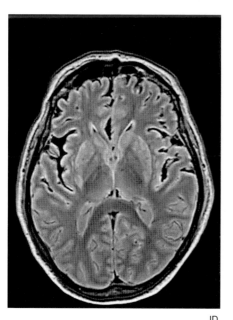

ID

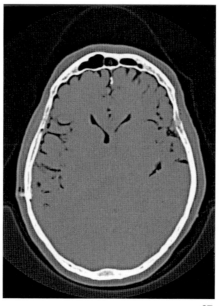

CT

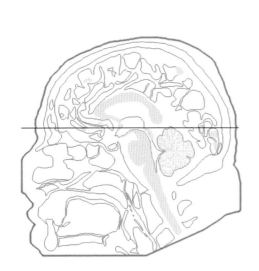

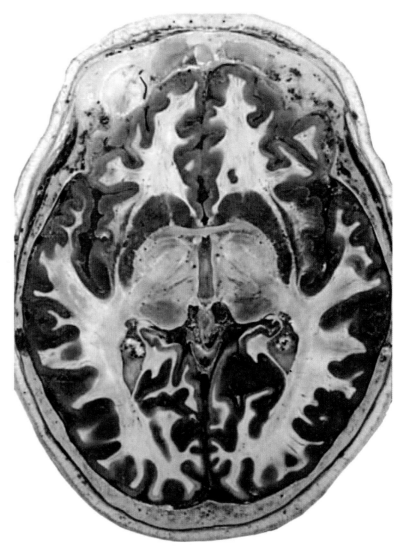

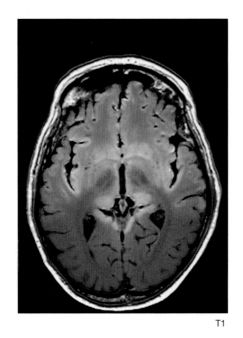

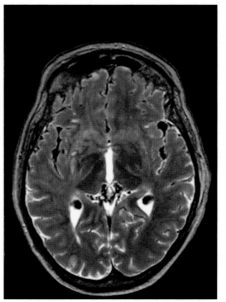

T1   T2

Axial   600

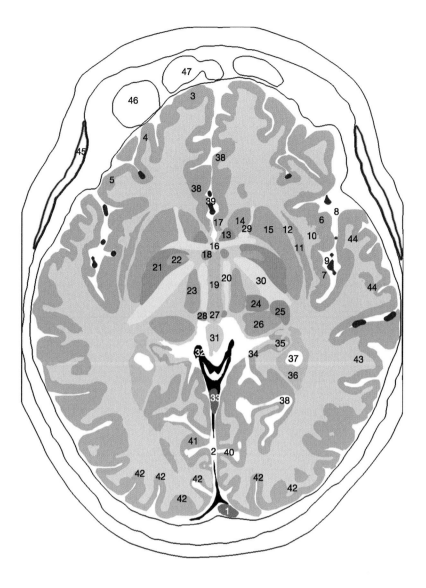

1 – Superior sagittal sinus
2 – Falx cerebri
3 – Superior frontal gyrus
4 – Middle frontal gyrus
5 – Inferior frontal gyrus
    (opercular part)
6 – Short insular gyri
7 – Long insular gyrus
8 – Lateral sulcus (Sylvius)
9 – Middle cerebral artery
10 – Extreme capsule
11 – Claustrum
12 – Capsula externa
13 – Nucleus accumbens
14 – Caudate nucleus
15 – Putamen
16 – Anterior commissure
17 – Area subcallosa
18 – Fornix column
19 – 3rd ventricle
20 – Mamillo-thalamic tract
21 – Globus pallidus pars externa
22 – Globus pallidus pars interna
23 – Centromedial thalamic nucleus
24 – Ventral posteromedial
    thalamic nucleus (VPM)
25 – Ventral posterolateral
    thalamic nucleus (VPL)
26 – Pulvinar nuclei of thalamus
27 – Suprapineal recess of third
    ventricle
28 – Nucleus habenulae
29 – Internal capsule (anterior limb)
30 – Internal capsule (posterior limb)
31 – Pineal body
32 – Tentorium cerebelli
33 – Straight sinus (sinus rectus)
34 – Parahippocampal gyrus
35 – Hippocampus
36 – Lateral ventricle (posterior horn)
37 – Choroid plexus
38 – Cingulate gyrus
39 – Anterior cerebral artery (ACA)
40 – Calcarine sulcus
41 – Striate area (Area striata)
42 – Occipital gyri
43 – Middle temporal gyrus
44 – Superior temporal gyrus
45 – Temporalis muscle and fascia
46 – Orbital roof (orbital roof of the
    frontal bone)
47 – Frontal sinus

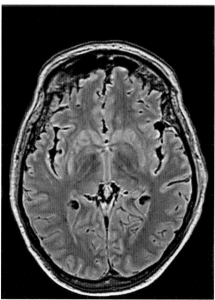

ID

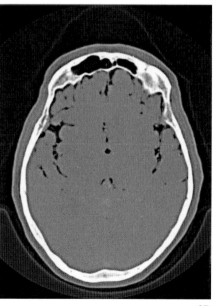

CT

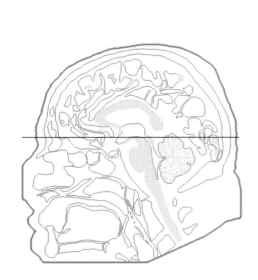

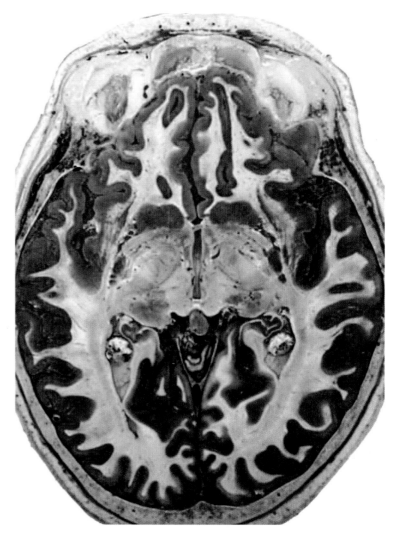

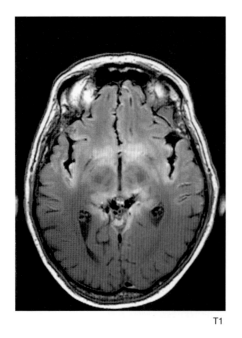
T1

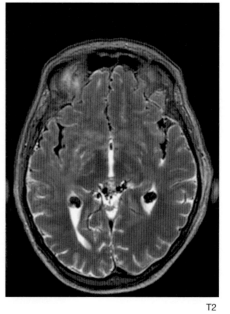
T2

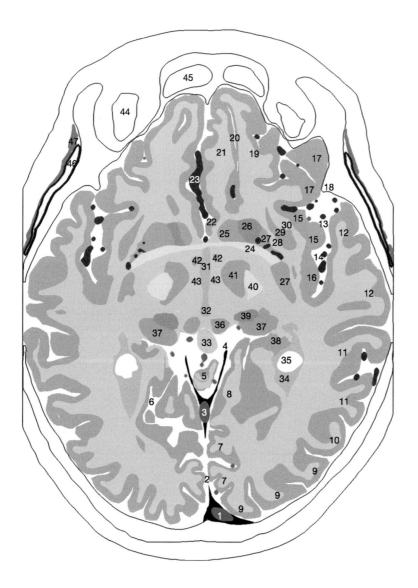

1 – Superior sagittal sinus
2 – Falx cerebri
3 – Sinus rectus
4 – Tentorium (medial margin)
5 – Cerebellar vermis
6 – Calcarine sulcus
7 – Cuneus
8 – Medial occipitotemporal gyrus
9 – Occipital gyri
10 – Inferior temporal gyrus
11 – Middle temporal gyrus
12 – Superior temporal gyrus
13 – Lateral sulcus (Sylvius)
14 – Middle cerebral artery
15 – Short insular gyri
16 – Long insular gyrus
17 – Inferior frontal gyrus
(frontal operculum)
18 – Sphenoid ridge
19 – Orbital gyri
20 – Olfactory sulcus
21 – Straight gyrus (gyrus rectus)
22 – Cingulate gyrus
23 – Anterior cerebral artery
24 – Anterior commissure
25 – Nucleus accumbens
26 – Head of caudate nucleus
27 – Putamen
28 – External capsule
29 – Claustrum
30 – Extreme capsule
31 – Third ventricle
32 – Suprapineal recess
of the third ventricle
33 – Pineal body
34 – Posterior horn of lateral ventricle
35 – Choroid plexus
36 – Superior colliculus
37 – Pulvinar nuclei of thalamus
38 – Hippocampus
39 – Lateral posterior nucleus
of thalamus
40 – Internal capsule (posterior limb)
41 – Ventral anterior nucleus
of thalamus (VL)
42 – Fornix columns
43 – Mamillo-thalamic tract
44 – Orbital roof (orbital roof of the
frontal bone)
45 – Frontal sinus
46 – Temporalis muscle
47 – Temporalis fascia

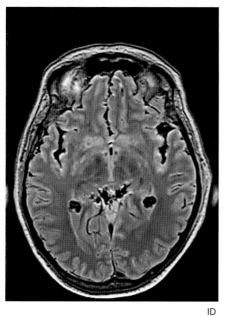

ID

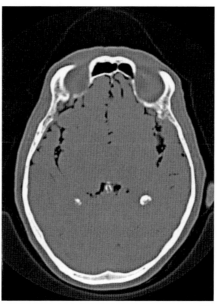

CT

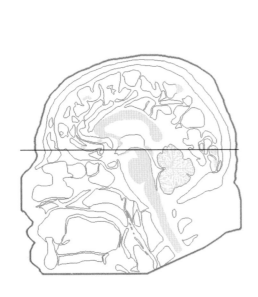

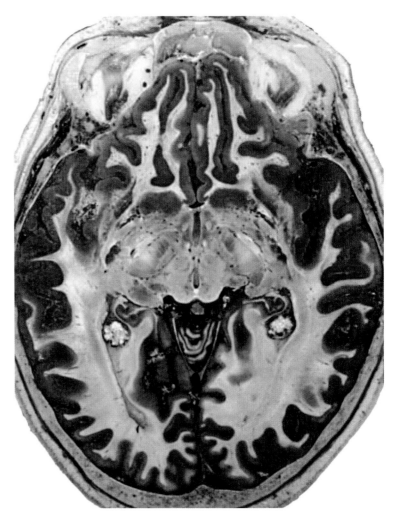

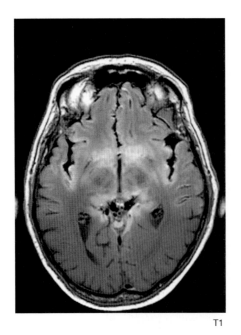

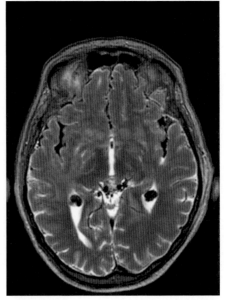

T1

T2

Axial   630

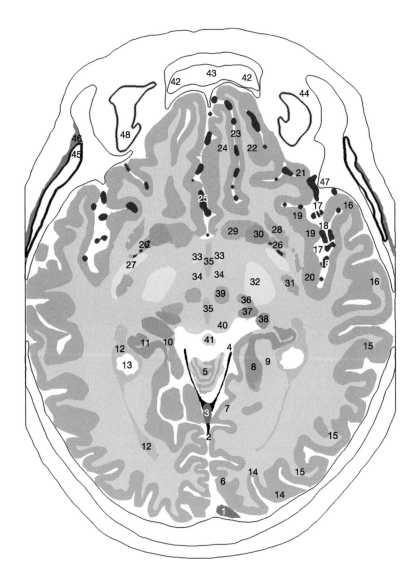

1 – Superior sagittal sinus
2 – Falx cerebri
3 – Straight sinus (sinus rectus)
4 – Tentorium (medial margin)
5 – Cerebellum
6 – Cuneus
7 – Medial occipitotemporal gyrus
8 – Collateral sulcus
9 – Lateral occipito-temporal gyrus
10 – Parahippocampal gyrus
11 – Hippocampus
12 – Lateral ventricle (posterior horn)
13 – Choroid plexus of lateral ventricle
14 – Occipital gyri
15 – Middle temporal gyrus
16 – Superior temporal gyrus
17 – Lateral sulcus (Sylvius)
18 – Middle cerebral artery
19 – Short insular gyri
20 – Long insular gyrus
21 – Inferior frontal gyrus
      (frontal operculum)
22 – Orbital gyri
23 – Olfactory sulcus
24 – Straight gyrus (gyrus rectus)
25 – Anterior cerebral artery
26 – Substantia perforata anterior
27 – Anterior commissure
28 – Claustrum
29 – Nucleus accumbens
30 – Head of caudate nucleus
31 – Putamen
32 – Internal capsule (posterior limb)
33 – Fornix columns
34 – Mamillo-thalamic tract
35 – Third ventricle
36 – Ventral posterolateral nucleus
      of thalamus (VPL)
37 – Medial geniculate body
38 – Lateral geniculate body
39 – Red nucleus
40 – Superior colliculus
41 – Pineal body
42 – Frontal sinus
43 – Ethmoidal cells
44 – Orbital roof (orbital part of
      the frontal bone)
45 – Temporalis muscle
46 – Temporalis fascia
47 – Sphenoid ridge

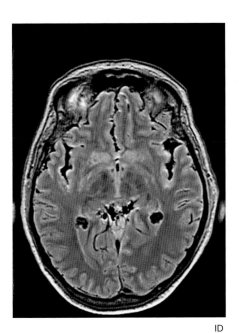

ID

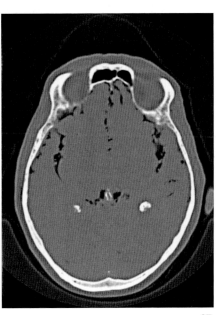

CT

Axial   630

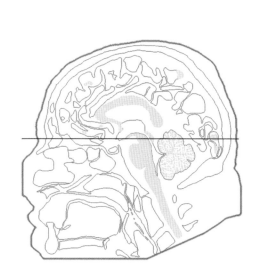

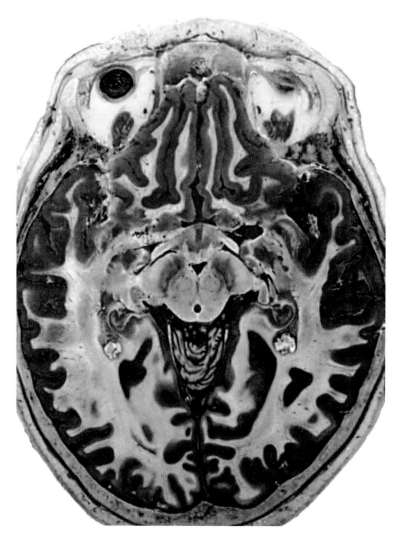

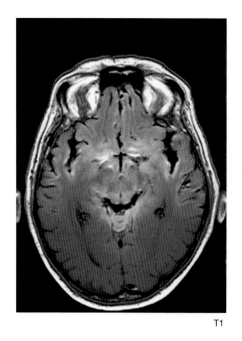

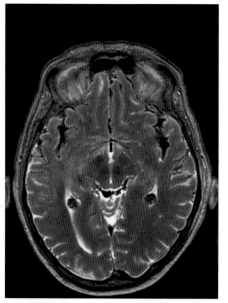

T1

T2

Axial   650

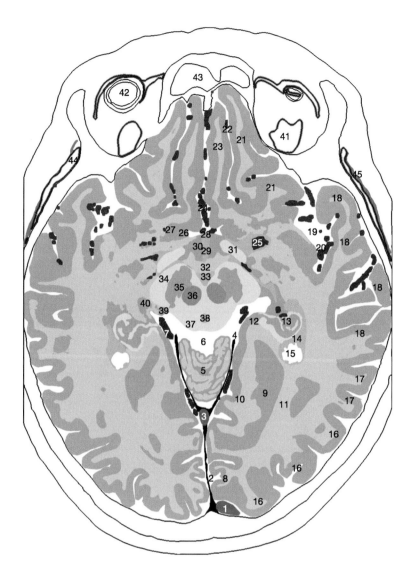

1 – Superior sagittal sinus
2 – Falx cerebri
3 – Straight sinus (sinus rectus)
4 – Tentorium cerebelli (medial margin)
5 – Cerebellum
6 – Perimesencephalic cistern
7 – Posterior cerebral artery
8 – Cuneus
9 – Collateral sulcus
10 – Medial occipitotemporal gyrus
11 – Lateral occipitotemporal gyrus
12 – Parahippocampal gyrus
13 – Hippocampus
14 – Lateral ventricle (posterior horn)
15 – Choroid plexus
16 – Occipital gyri
17 – Middle temporal gyrus
18 – Superior temporal gyrus
19 – Lateral sulcus (Sylvius)
20 – Middle cerebral artery
21 – Orbital gyri
22 – Olfactory sulcus
23 – Straight gyrus (gyrus rectus)
24 – Anterior cerebral artery
25 – Internal carotid artery
26 – Nucleus accumbens
27 – Head of caudate nucleus
28 – Lamina terminalis
29 – Third ventricle (supraoptic recess)
30 – Hypothalamus
31 – Optic tract
32 – Mamillary bodies
33 – Interpeduncular fossa and cistern
34 – Cerebral peduncle
35 – Substantia nigra
36 – Red nucleus
37 – Inferior colliculus
38 – Cerebral aqueduct
39 – Medial geniculate body
40 – Lateral geniculate body
41 – Rectus superior muscle
42 – Eyeball
43 – Ethmoidal cells
44 – Temporalis muscle
45 – Temporalis fascia

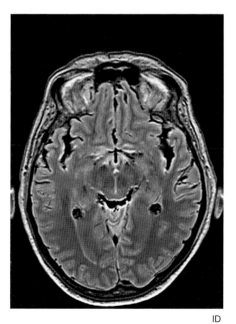

ID

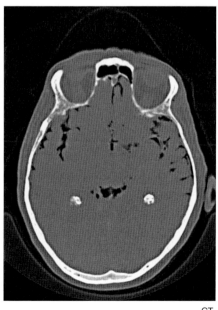

CT

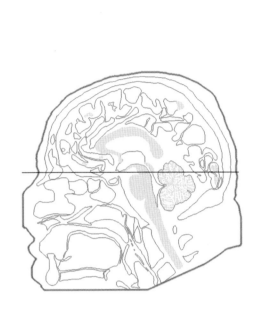

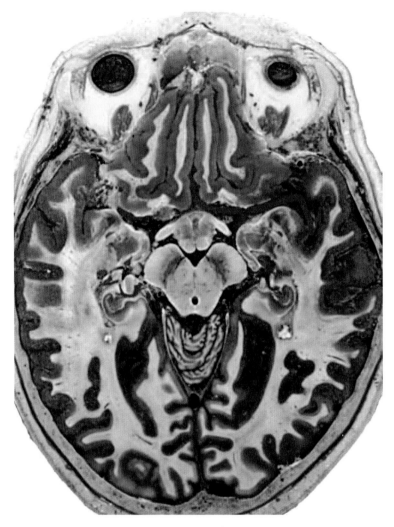

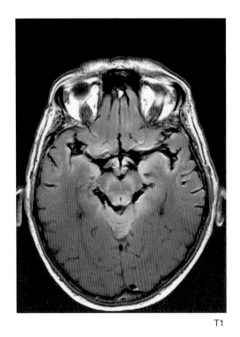

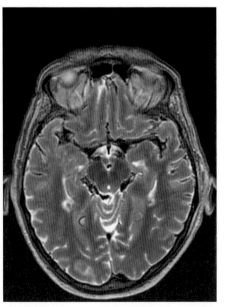

T1

T2

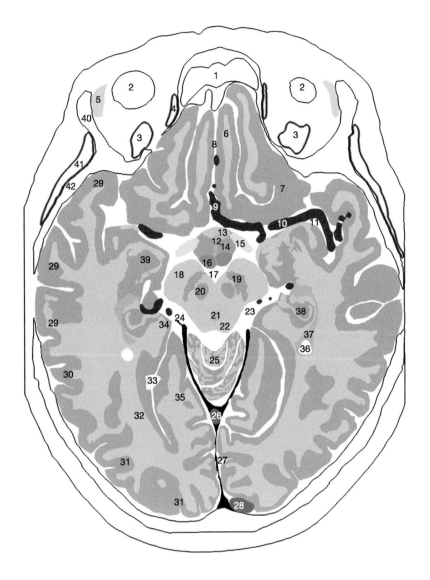

1 – Ethmoidal cells
2 – Eyeball
3 – Superior rectus muscle
4 – Medial rectus muscle
5 – Lacrimal gland
6 – Straight gyrus (gyrus rectus)
7 – Orbital gyri
8 – Interhemispheric fissure
9 – Anterior cerebral artery
10 – Middle cerebral artery
11 – Lateral sulcus (Sylvius)
12 – Third ventricle
      (supraoptic recess)
13 – Lamina terminalis
14 – Hypothalamus
15 – Optic tract
16 – Mammillary body
17 – Interpeduncular fossa and cistern
18 – Cerebral peduncle
19 – Substantia nigra
20 – Red nucleus
21 – Cerebral aqueduct
22 – Superior colliculus
23 – Perimesencephalic cistern
24 – Tentorium cerebelli
25 – Cerebellum (central lobule)
26 – Straight sinus (sinus rectus)
27 – Falx cerebri
28 – Superior sagittal sinus
29 – Superior temporal gyrus
30 – Middle temporal gyrus
31 – Occipital gyri
32 – Lateral occipitotemporal gyrus
33 – Collateral sulcus
34 – Parahippocampal gyrus
35 – Medial occipito-temporal gyrus
36 – Choroid plexus
37 – Lateral ventricle
38 – Hippocampus
39 – Amygdaloid body
40 – Greater sphenoid wing
41 – Temporalis muscle
42 – Temporal bone (squama)

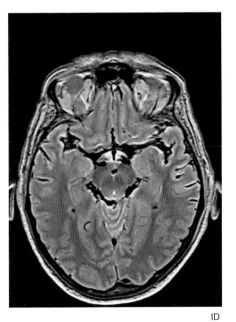

ID

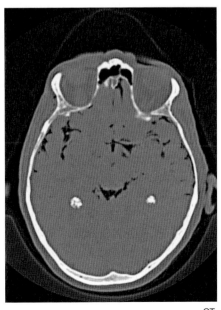

CT

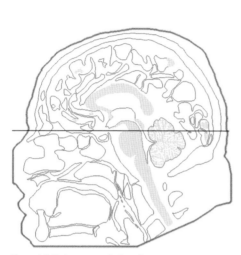

For a detail view see end of section

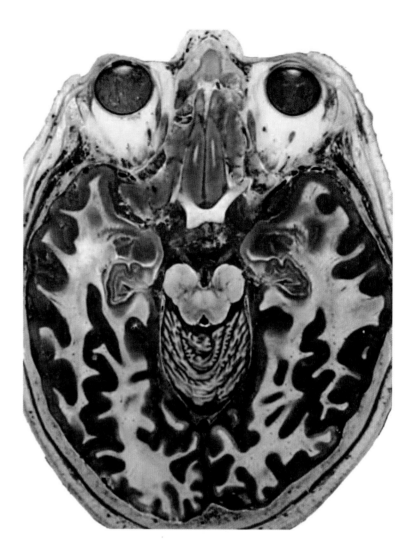

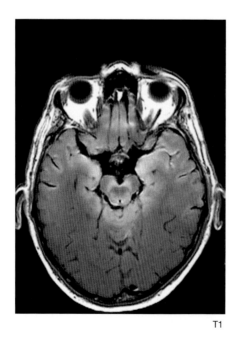

T1

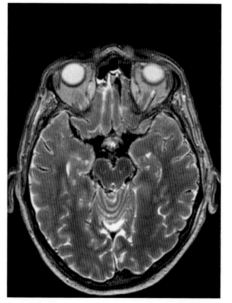

T2

Axial   691

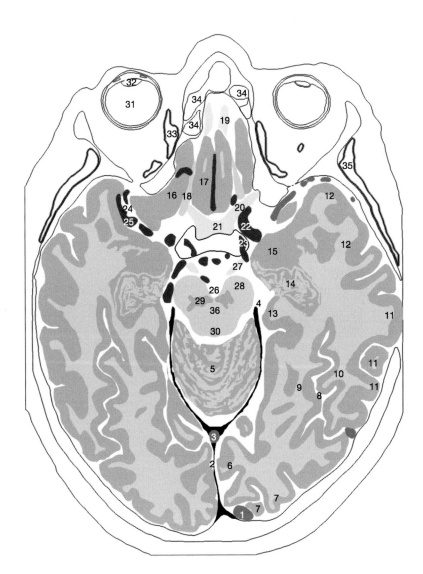

1 – Superior sagittal sinus
2 – Falx cerebri
3 – Straight sinus (sinus rectus)
4 – Tentorium cerebelli
5 – Cerebellum
6 – Cuneus
7 – Occipital gyri
8 – Collateral sulcus
9 – Medial occipitotemporal gyrus
10 – Lateral occipitotemporal gyrus
11 – Middle temporal gyrus
12 – Superior temporal gyrus
13 – Parahippocampal gyrus
14 – Hippocampus
15 – Amygdaloid body
16 – Orbital gyri
17 – Straight gyrus (gyrus rectus)
18 – Olfactory tract
19 – Olfactory bulb
20 – Optic nerve (CN II)
21 – Optic chiasm
22 – Internal carotid artery
23 – Posterior communicating artery
24 – Lateral sulcus (Sylvius)
25 – Middle cerebral artery
26 – Interpeduncular fossa and cistern
27 – Occulomotor nerve (CN III)
28 – Cerebral peduncle
29 – Substantia nigra
30 – Cerebral aqueduct
31 – Eyeball (vitreous chamber)
32 – Lens
33 – Medial rectus muscle
34 – Ethmoidal cells
35 – Temporalis muscle
36 – Decussation of the superior cerebellar peduncles

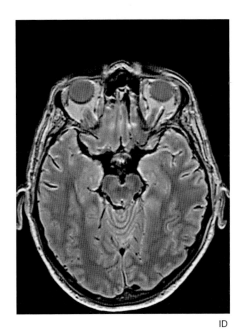

ID

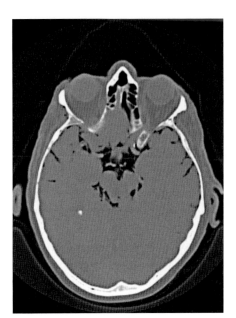

CT

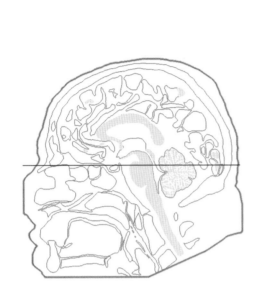

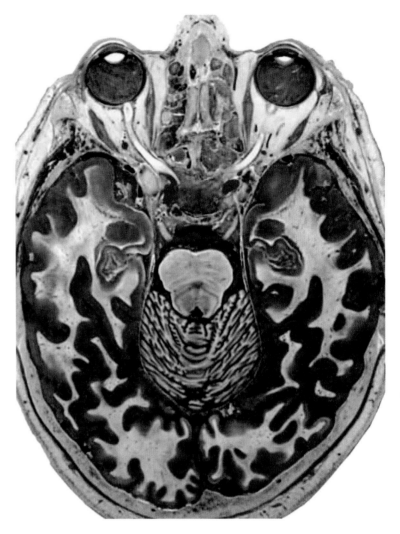

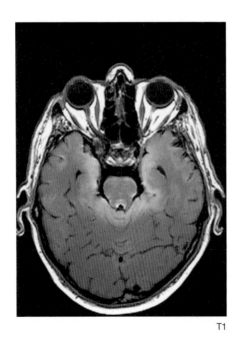

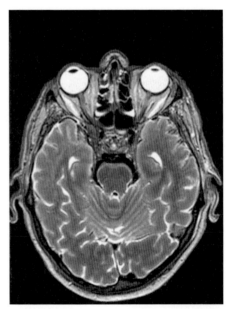

T1

T2

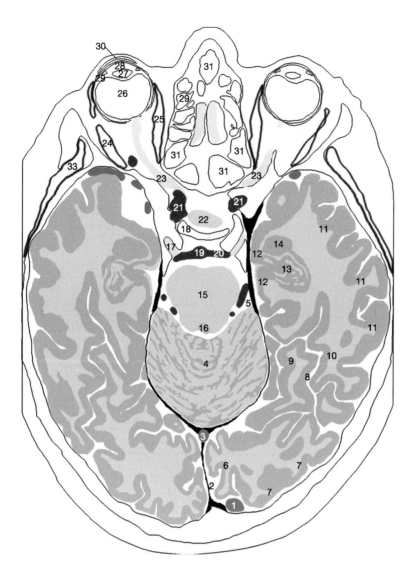

1 – Superior sagittal sinus
2 – Falx cerebri
3 – Straight sinus (sinus rectus)
4 – Cerebellum
5 – Tentorium cerebelli
6 – Cuneus
7 – Occipital gyri
8 – Collateral sulcus
9 – Medial occipitotemporal gyrus
10 – Lateral occipitotemporal gyrus
11 – Middle temporal gyrus
12 – Parahippocampal gyrus
13 – Hippocampus
14 – Amygdaloid body
15 – Upper pons
16 – Cerebral aqueduct
17 – Occulomotor nerve (CN III)
18 – Posterior clinoid process
19 – Basilar artery
20 – Superior cerebellar artery
21 – Internal carotid artery
22 – Pituitary gland
23 – Optic nerve (CN II)
24 – Lateral rectus muscle
25 – Medial rectus muscle
26 – Eyeball (vitreous chamber)
27 – Lens
28 – Anterior chamber of the eye
29 – Ciliary body
30 – Upper tarsus
31 – Ethmoidal cells
32 – Nasal bone
33 – Temporalis muscle

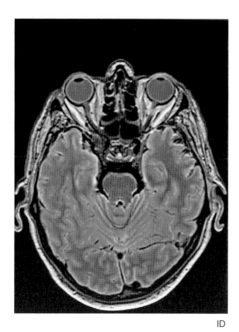

ID

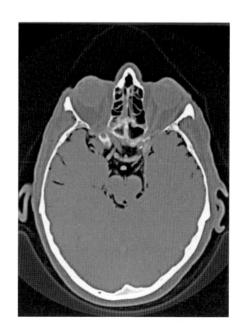

CT

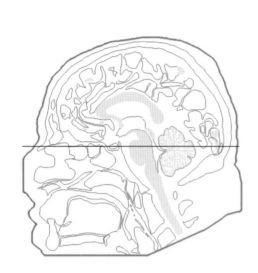

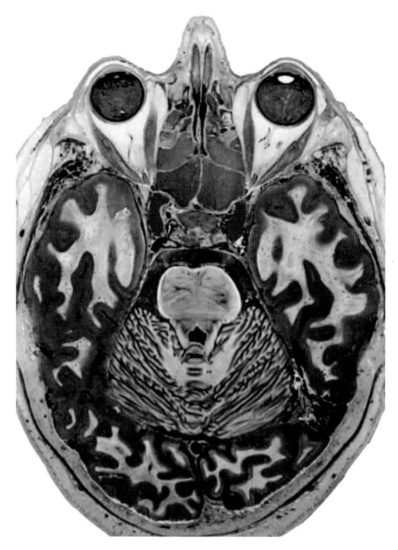

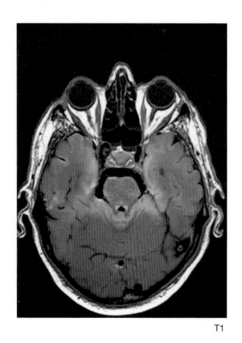

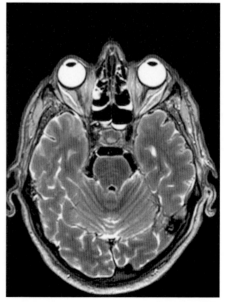

T1

T2

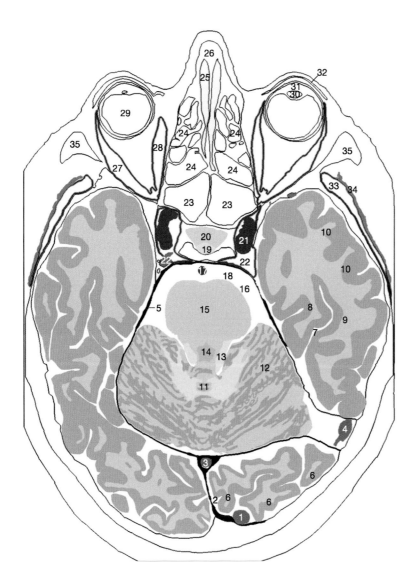

1 – Superior sagittal sinus
2 – Falx cerebri
3 – Straight sinus (sinus rectus)
4 – Sigmoid sinus
5 – Tentorium cerebelli
6 – Occipital gyri
7 – Collateral sulcus
8 – Medial occipitotemporal gyrus
9 – Lateral occipitotemporal gyrus
10 – Inferior temporal gyrus
11 – Cerebellum (culmen)
12 – Cerebellar hemisphere
13 – Superior cerebellar peduncle
14 – Fourth ventricle
15 – Pons
16 – Pontocerebellar cistern
17 – Basilar artery
18 – Clivus
19 – Pituitary gland (posterior lobe)
20 – Pituitary gland (anterior lobe)
21 – Internal carotid artery
22 – Cavernous sinus
23 – Sphenoid sinus
24 – Ethmoidal cells
25 – Superior nasal concha
26 – Nasal bone
27 – Lateral rectus muscle
28 – Medial rectus muscle
29 – Eyeball (vitreous chamber)
30 – Lens
31 – Anterior chamber of the eye
32 – Upper tarsus
33 – Temporalis muscle
34 – Temporalis fascia
35 – Zygomatic arch

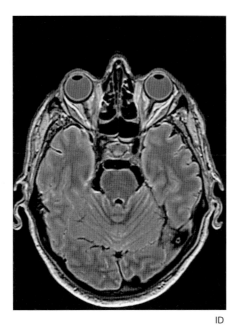

ID

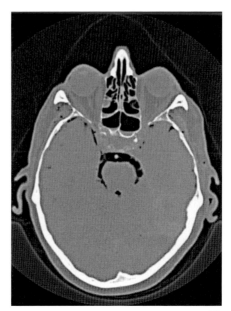

CT

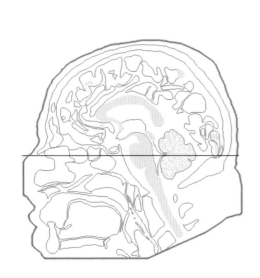

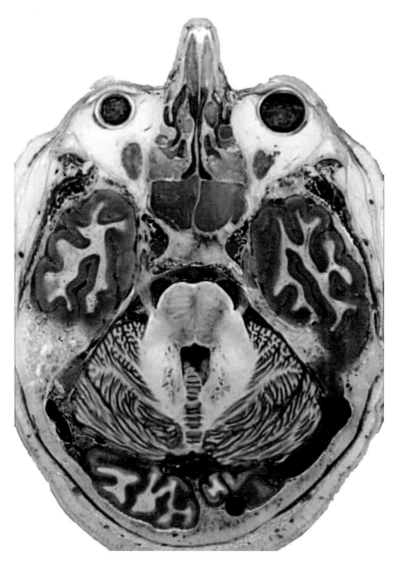

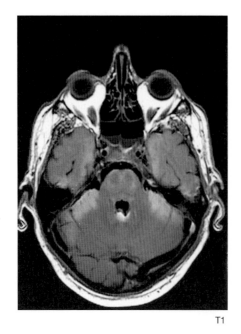 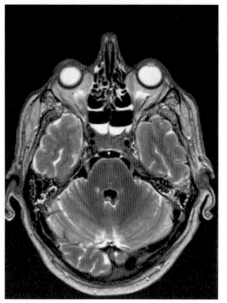

T1　　　　　　　　　　　　T2

Axial　780

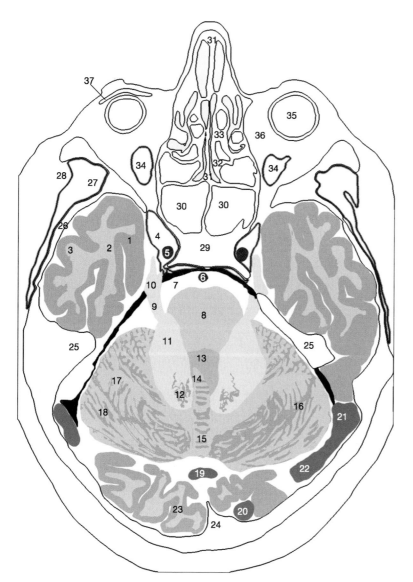

1 – Parahippocampal gyrus
2 – Lateral occipito-temporal gyrus
3 – Inferior temporal gyrus
4 – Cavernous sinus
5 – Internal carotid artery
6 – Basilar artery
7 – Pontocerebellar cistern
8 – Pons
9 – Trigeminal nerve (CN V)
10 – Ganglion of the trigeminal nerve (Gasser)
11 – Middle cerebellar peduncle
12 – Dentate nucleus
13 – Fourth ventricle
14 – Nodulus of the cerebellum
15 – Tuber of the cerebellum
16 – Horizontal fissure of the cerebellum
17 – Superior semilunar lobule
      of the cerebellum
18 – Inferior semilunar lobule
      of the cerebellum
19 – Straight sinus (sinus rectus)
20 – Superior sagittal sinus
21 – Sigmoid sinus
22 – Transverse sinus
23 – Occipital gyri
24 – Internal occipital protuberance
25 – Petrous bone
26 – Temporal bone (squama)
27 – Temporalis muscle
      in the infratemporal fossa
28 – Zygomatic arch
29 – Body of the sphenoid bone
30 – Sphenoid sinus
31 – Nasal septum
32 – Superior nasal concha
33 – Middle nasal concha
34 – Inferior rectus muscle
35 – Eyeball
36 – Orbital fat body
37 – Inferior tarsus

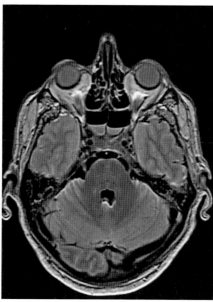

ID

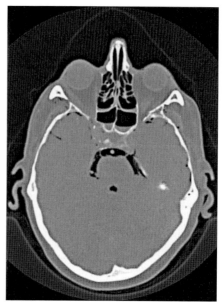

CT

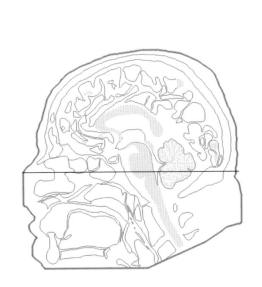

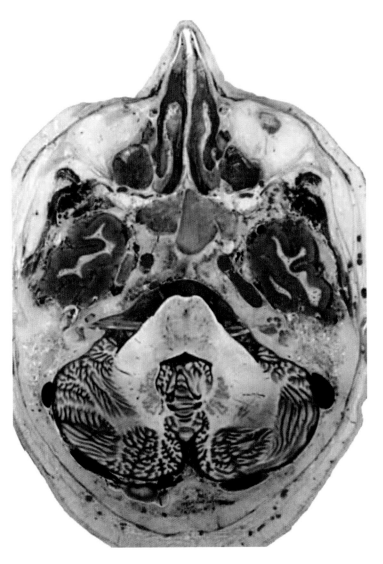

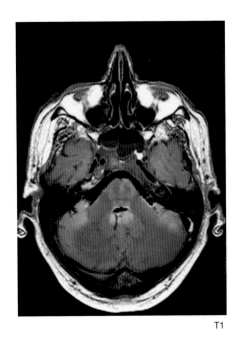

T1

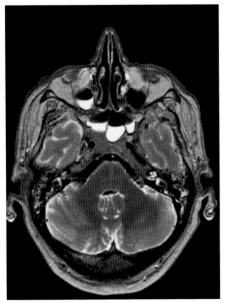

T2

Axial   830

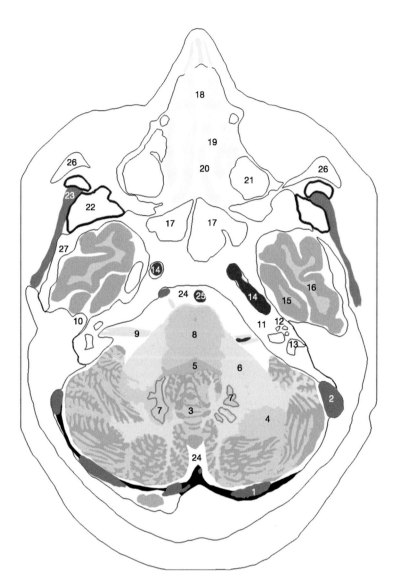

1 – Transverse sinus
2 – Sigmoid sinus
3 – Vermis of cerebellum
4 – Cerebellar hemisphere
5 – Fourth ventricle
6 – Inferior cerebellar peduncle
7 – Dentate nucleus
8 – Medulla oblongata
9 – Vestibulo-cochlear nerve
      (CN VIII)
10 – Internal acoustic meatus
11 – Petrous bone
12 – Semicircular canals
13 – Cochlea
14 – Internal carotid artery
15 – Lateral occipitotemporal gyrus
16 – Inferior temporal gyrus
17 – Sphenoid sinus
18 – Nasal septum
19 – Middle nasal concha
20 – Nasal cavity
21 – Maxillary sinus
22 – Temporalis muscle
23 – Temporalis fascia
24 – Cerebellomedullary cistern
      (Cisterna magna)
25 – Basilar artery
26 – Zygomatic bone
27 – Temporal bone (squama)

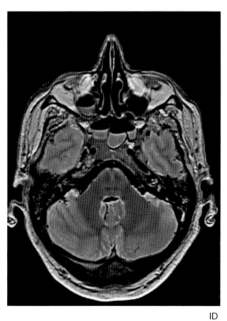

ID

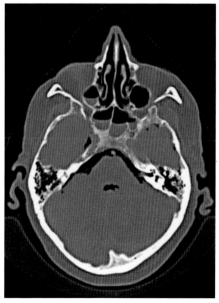

CT

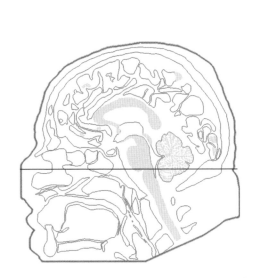

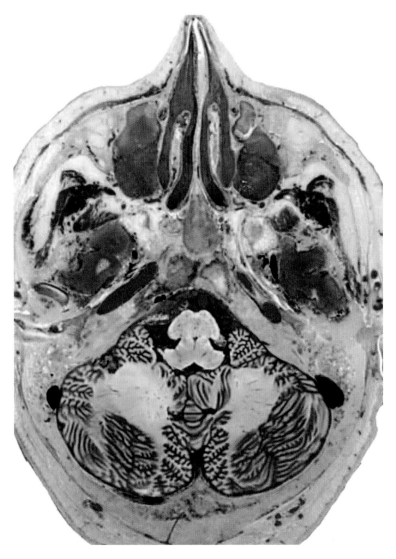

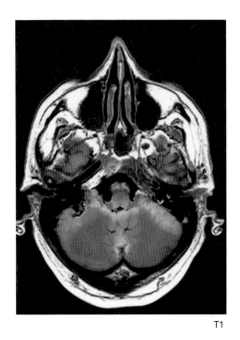

T1

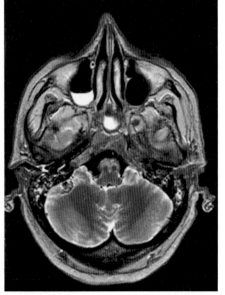

T2

Axial   858

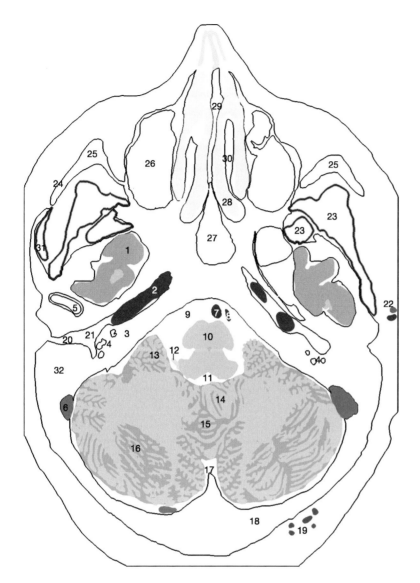

1 – Lateral occipito-temporal gyrus
2 – Internal carotid artery
3 – Petrous bone
4 – Internal ear
5 – Temporo-mandibular joint
6 – Sigmoid sinus
7 – Basilar artery
8 – Anterior inferior cerebellar artery (AICA)
9 – Pontocerebellar cistern
10 – Pons
11 – Fourth ventricle
12 – Vestibulo-cochlear nerve (CN VIII)
13 – Flocculus
14 – Cerebellar tonsil
15 – Cerebellar vermis
16 – Cerebellar hemisphere
17 – Internal occipital protuberance
18 – Occipital bone (squama)
19 – Branches of the occipital artery
20 – External auditory canal
21 – Middle ear
22 – Superficial temporal artery and vein
23 – Temporalis muscle
24 – Zygomatic arch
25 – Zygomatic bone
26 – Maxillary sinus
27 – Sphenoid sinus
28 – Nasal cavity
29 – Nasal septum
30 – Middle nasal concha
31 – Masseter muscle
32 – Mastoid process

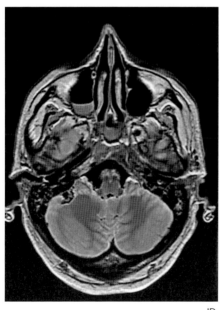

ID

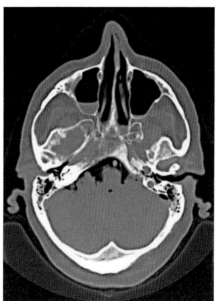

CT

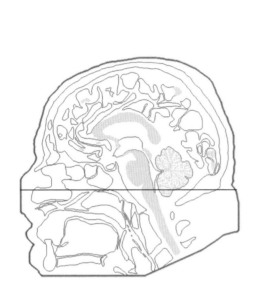

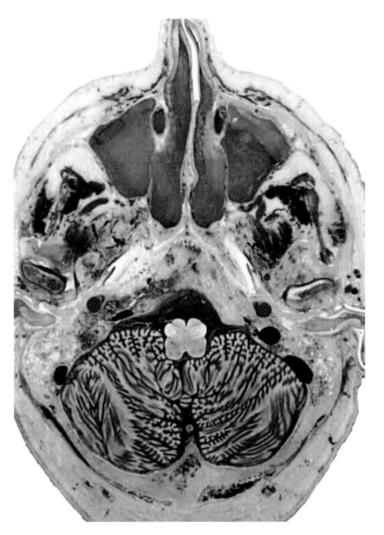

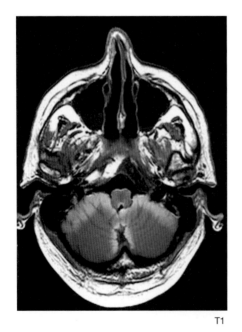

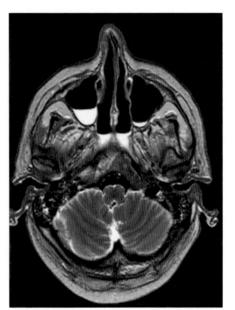

T1

T2

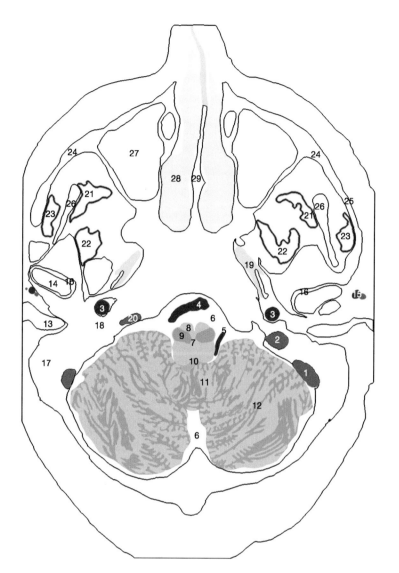

1 – Sigmoid sinus
2 – Bulb of jugular vein
3 – Internal carotid artery
4 – Vertebral artery
5 – Posterior inferior cerebellar artery (PICA)
6 – Cerebellomedullary cistern (Cisterna magna)
7 – Medulla oblongata
8 – Pyramid
9 – Olive
10 – Fourth ventricle
11 – Cerebellar tonsil
12 – Cerebellar hemisphere
13 – External auditory canal
14 – Head of mandible
15 – Superficial temporal artery
16 – Temporomandibular joint
17 – Mastoid process
18 – Petrous bone
19 – Pharyngotympanic (auditory) tube (Eustachio)
20 – Inferior petrosal sinus
21 – Temporalis muscle
22 – Lateral pterygoid muscle
23 – Masseter muscle
24 – Zygomatic bone
25 – Zygomatic arch
26 – Mandible (coronoid process)
27 – Maxillary sinus
28 – Nasal cavity
29 – Nasal septum

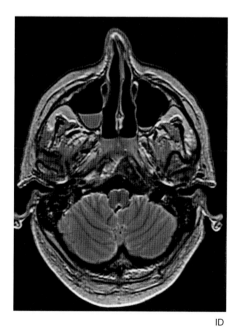

ID

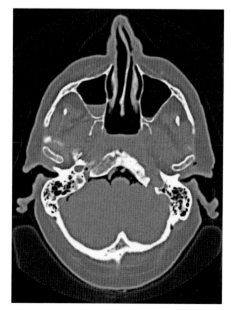

CT

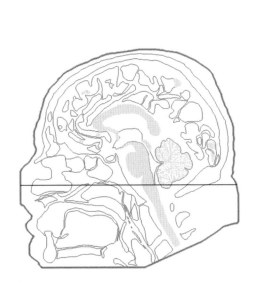

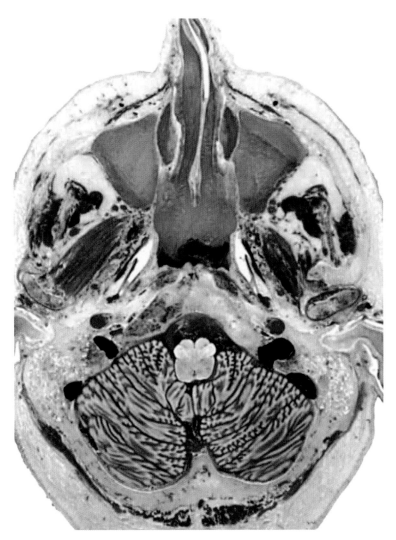

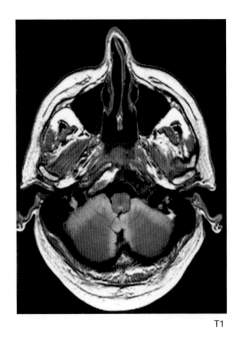

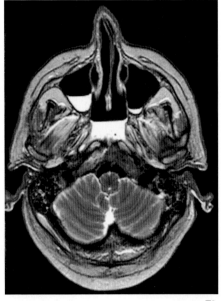

T1

T2

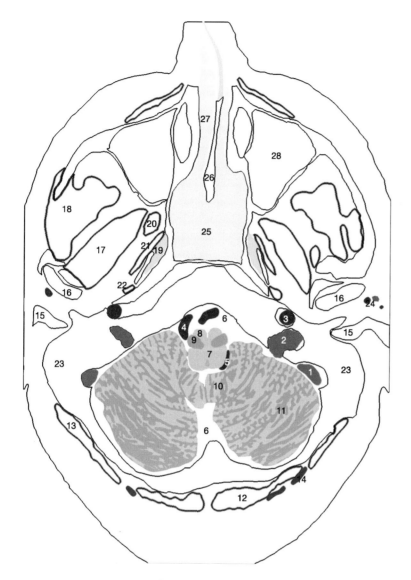

1 – Sigmoid sinus
2 – Bulb of jugular vein
3 – Internal carotid artery
4 – Vertebral artery
5 – Posterior inferior cerebellar artery (PICA)
6 – Cerebellomedullary cistern (Cisterna magna)
7 – Medulla oblongata
8 – Pyramid
9 – Olive
10 – Cerebellar tonsil
11 – Cerebellar hemisphere
12 – Semispinalis capitis muscle
13 – Trapezius muscle
14 – Occipital artery
15 – External auditory canal
16 – Head of mandible
17 – Medial pterygoid muscle
18 – Lateral pterygoid muscle
19 – Pharyngotympanic (auditory) tube (Eustachio)
20 – Tensor veli palatini muscle
21 – Levator veli palatini muscle
22 – Salpingopahryngeus muscle
23 – Mastoid process
24 – Superficial temporal artery and vein
25 – Rhinopharynx
26 – Nasal septum
27 – Nasal cavity
28 – Maxillary sinus

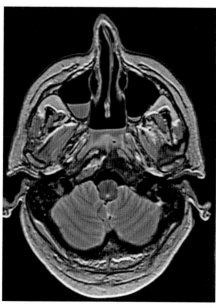

ID

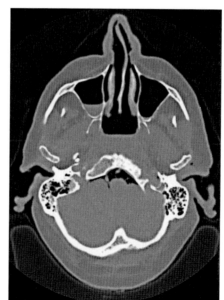

CT

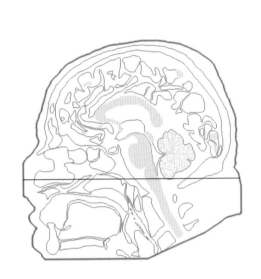

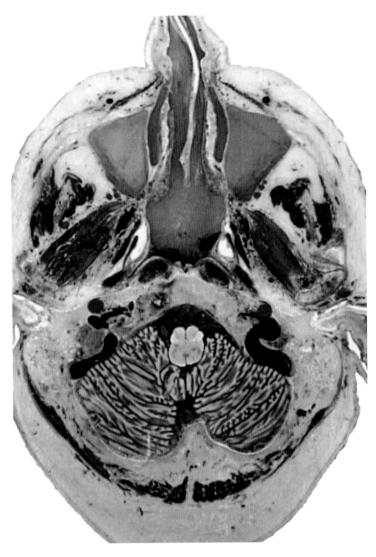

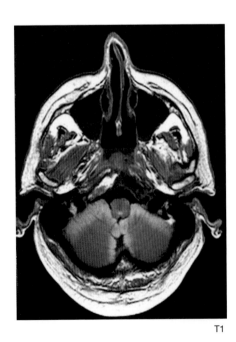

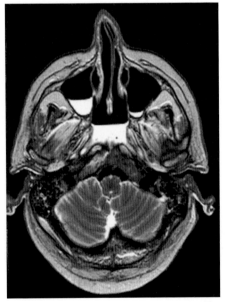

T1

T2

Axial   944

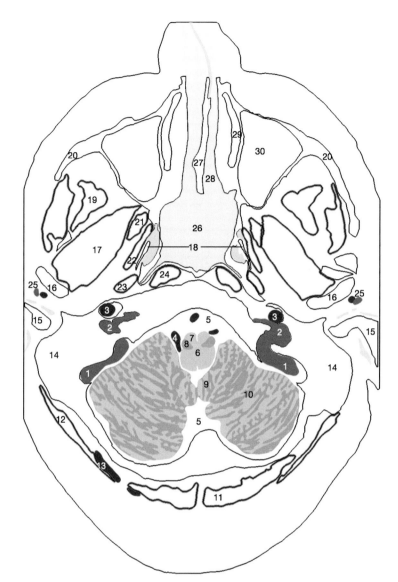

1 – Sigmoid sinus
2 – Bulb of jugular vein
3 – Internal carotid artery
4 – Vertebral artery
5 – Cerebellomedullary cistern
    (Cisterna magna)
6 – Medulla oblongata
7 – Pyramid
8 – Olive
9 – Cerebellar tonsil
10 – Cerebellar hemisphere
11 – Semispinalis capitis
12 – Trapezius muscle
13 – Occipital artery
14 – Mastoid process
15 – External auditory canal
16 – Head of mandible
17 – Medial pterygoid muscle
18 – Pharyngotympanic (auditory) tube
    (Eustachio)
19 – Lateral pterygoid muscle
20 – Zygomatic arch
21 – Tensor veli palatini muscle
22 – Levator veli palatini muscle
23 – Salpyngopharyngeus muscle
24 – Longus capitis muscle
25 – Superficial temporal artery and vein
26 – Rhinopharynx
27 – Nasal septum
28 – Nasal cavity
29 – Inferior nasal concha
30 – Maxillary sinus

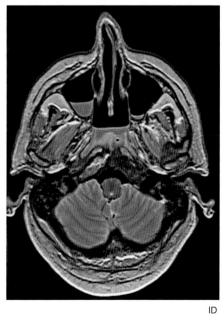

ID

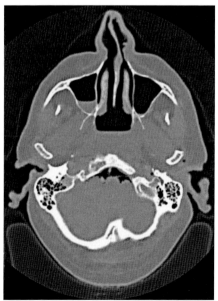

CT

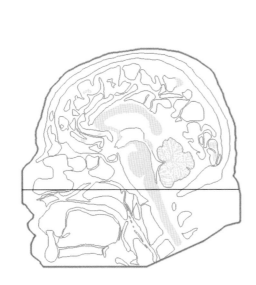

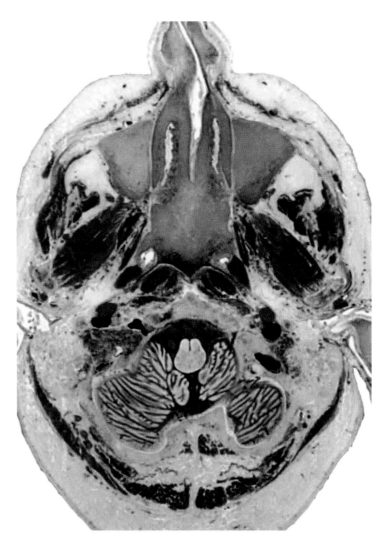

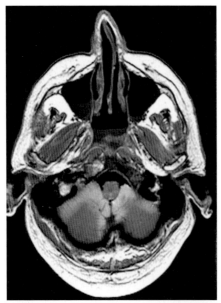

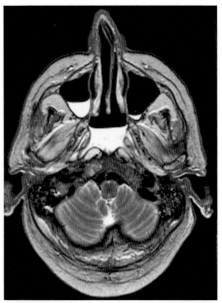

T1

T2

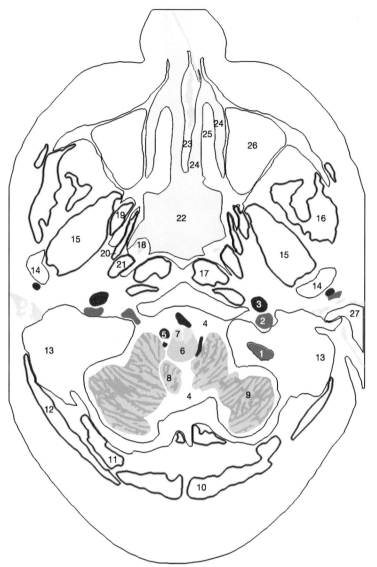

1 – Sigmoid sinus
2 – Bulb of jugular vein
3 – Internal carotid artery
4 – Cerebellomedullary cistern (Cisterna magna)
5 – Vertebral artery
6 – Medulla oblongata
7 – Pyramid
8 – Cerebellar tonsil
9 – Cerebellar hemisphere
10 – Semispinalis capitis muscle
11 – Splenius capitis muscle
12 – Trapezius muscle
13 – Mastoid process
14 – Mandible
15 – Medial pterygoid muscle
16 – Lateral pterygoid muscle
17 – Longus capitis muscle
18 – Pharyngotympanic (auditory) tube (Eustachio)
19 – Tensor veli palatini muscle
20 – Levator veli palatini muscle
21 – Salpyngopharyngeus muscle
22 – Rhinopharynx
23 – Nasal septum
24 – Nasal cavity
25 – Inferior nasal concha
26 – Maxiallary sinus
27 – External auditory canal

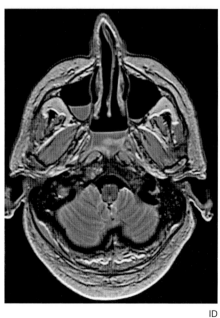

ID

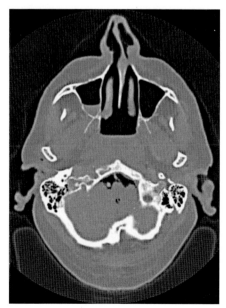

CT

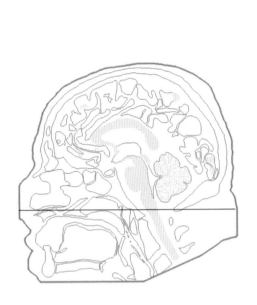

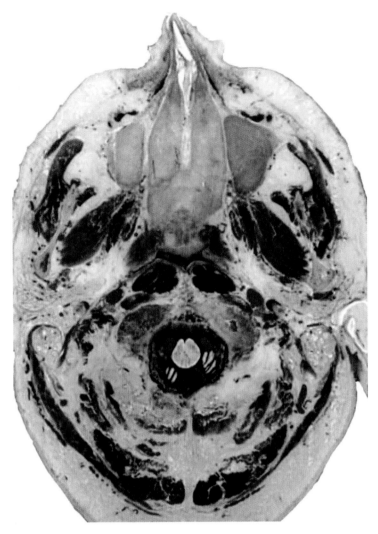

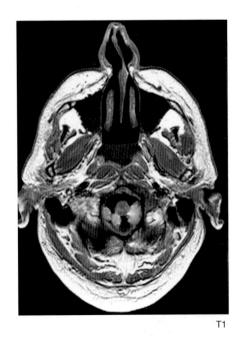

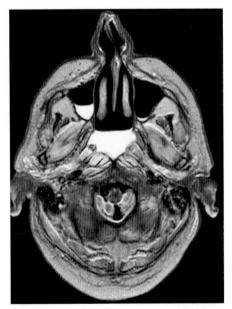

T1

T2

Axial 1009

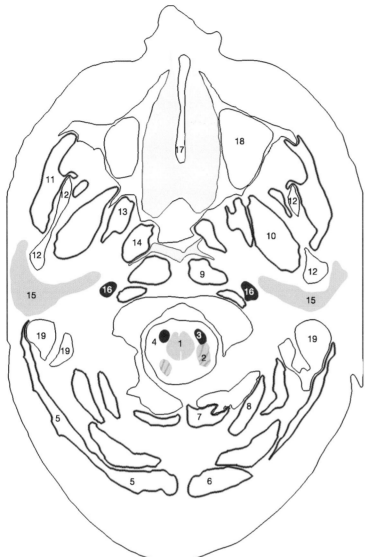

1 – Medulla oblongata
2 – Cerebellar tonsil
3 – Vertebral artery
4 – Foramen magnum
5 – Trapezius muscle
6 – Semispinalis capitis muscle
7 – Rectus capitis posterior
    minor muscle
8 – Rectus capitis posterior
    major muscle
9 – Longus capitis muscle
10 – Medial pterygoid muscle
11 – Masseter muscle
12 – Mandible (ramus)
13 – Tensor veli palatini muscle
14 – Levator veli palatini muscle
15 – Parotid gland
16 – Internal carotid artery
11 – Nasal cavity
17 – Nasal septum
18 – Maxillary sinus
19 – Mastoid process

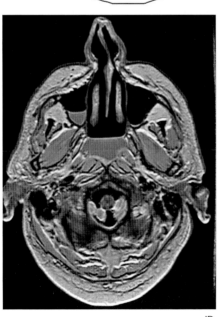

ID

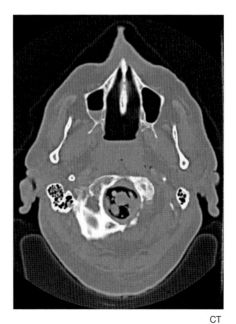

CT

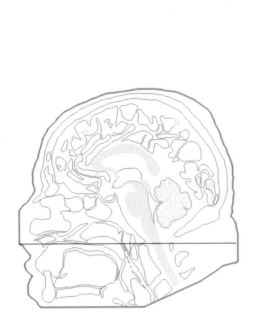

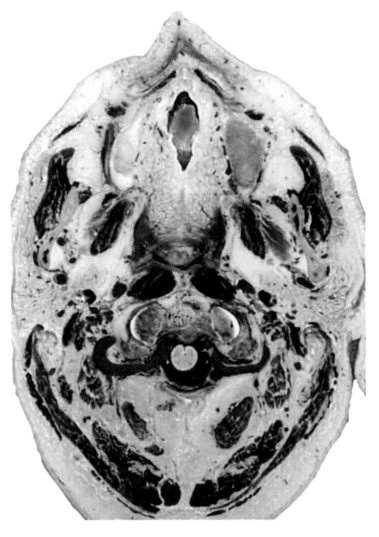

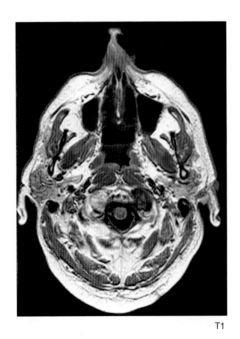

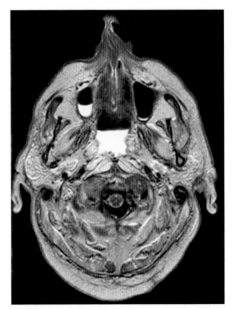

T1

T2

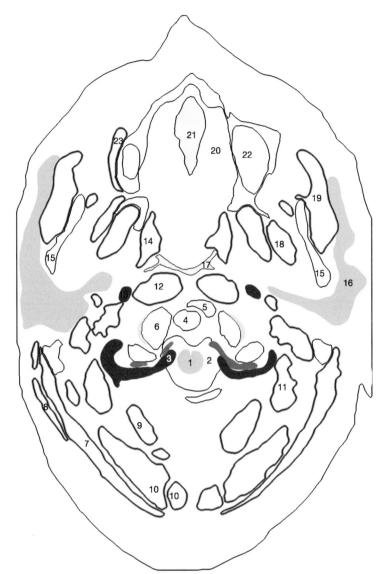

1 – Medulla oblongata
2 – Foramen magnum
3 – Vertebral artery
4 – Dens of axis
5 – Anterior arch of atlas
6 – Atlantooccipital joint
7 – Splenius caapitis muscle
8 – Trapezius muscle
9 – Rectus capitis posterior
  major muscle
10 – Semispinalis capitis muscle
11 – Obliquus capitis superior muscle
12 – Longus capitis muscle
13 – Internal carotid artery
14 – Tenosor veli palatini muscle
15 – Mandible
16 – Parotid gland
17 – Pharynx
18 – Medial pterygoid muscle
19 – Masseter muscle
20 – Hard palate
21 – Oral cavity
22 – Maxillary sinus
23 – Buccinator muscle

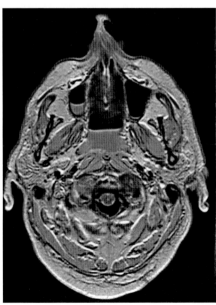

ID

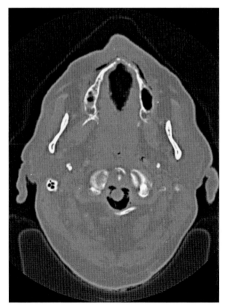

CT

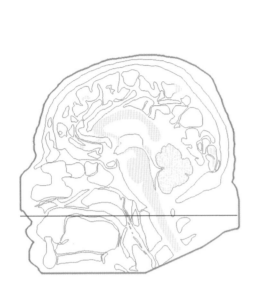

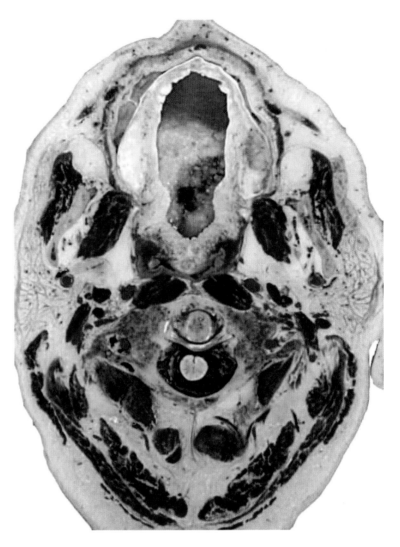

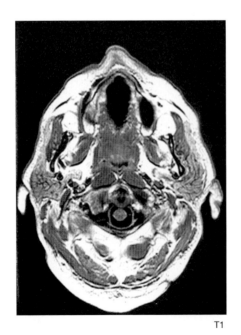

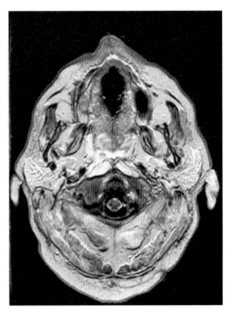

T1

T2

Axial   1080

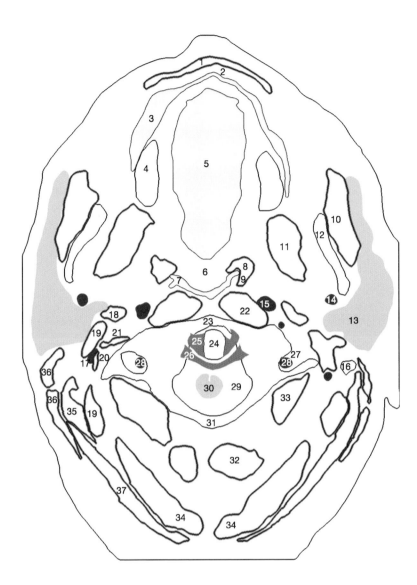

1 – Orbicularis oris muscle
2 – Upper lip
3 – Oral vestibulum
4 – Maxilla, alveolar process
5 – Hard palate
6 – Soft palate
7 – Oropharynx
8 – Tensor veli palatini muscle
9 – Levator veli palatini muscle
10 – Massetter muscle
11 – Medial pterygoid muscle
12 – Mandible (ramus)
13 – Parotid gland
14 – Maxillary artery
15 – Internal carotid artery
16 – Mastoid process
17 – Stylomastoid artery
18 – Stylohyoid muscle
19 – Digastric muscle (posterior belly)
20 – Styloglossus muscle
21 – Stylopharingeus muscle
22 – Longus capitis muscle
23 – Atlas (anterior arch)
24 – Dens of axis
25 – Alar ligament
26 – Transverse ligament of atlas
27 – Foramen transversarium
28 – Vertebral artery
29 – Spinal canal
30 – Medula oblongata
31 – Posterior arch of the atlas
32 – Rectus capitis posterior
        minor muscle
33 – Rectus capitis posterior
        major muscle
34 – Semispinalis capitis muscle
35 – Longissimus capitis muscle
36 – Sternocleidomastoid muscle
37 – Trapezius muscle

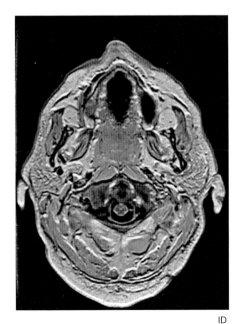

ID

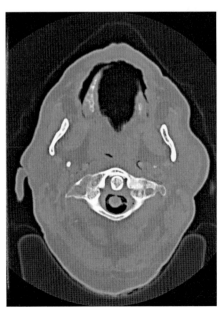

CT

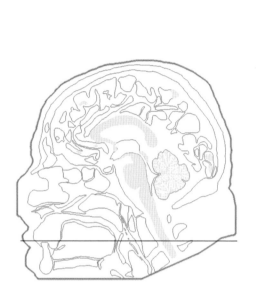

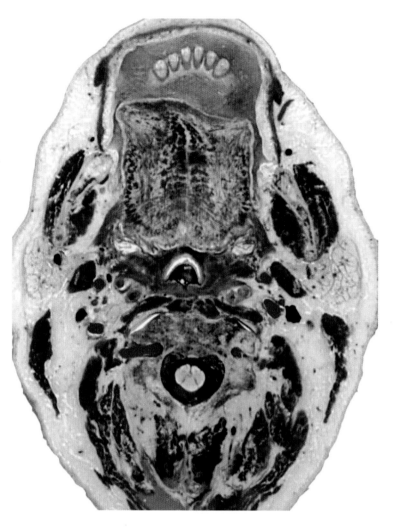

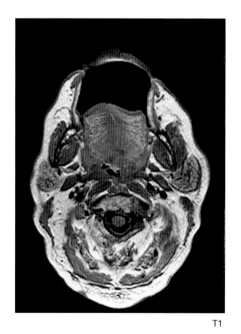

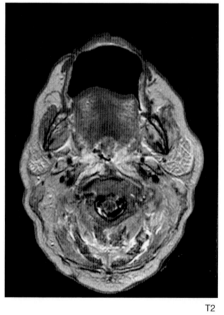

T1

T2

Axial   1206

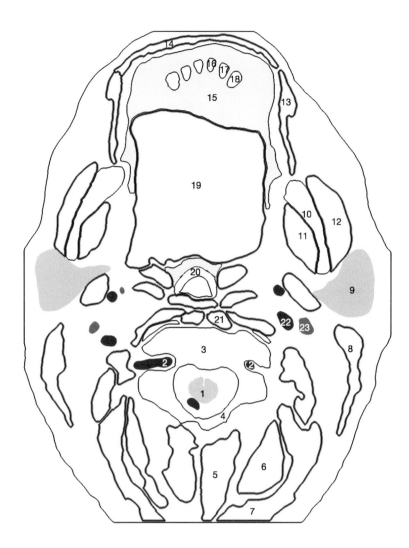

1 – Spinal cord
2 – Vertebral artery
3 – Body of axis
4 – Arch of axis
5 – Rectus capitis posterior
    minor muscle
6 – Rectus capitis posterior
    major muscle
7 – Semispinalis capitis
    muscle
8 – Sternocleidomastoid
    muscle
9 – Parotid gland
10 – Mandible
11 – Medial pterygoid muscle
12 – Masseter muscle
13 – Buccinator muscle
14 – Orbicularis oris muscle
15 – Oral cavity
16 – Left central inferior
     incisor tooth
17 – Left lateral inferior
     incisor tooth
18 – Left inferior canine tooth
19 – Tongue
20 – Epiglottis
21 – Longus capitis muscle
22 – Internal carotid artery
23 – Internal jugular vein

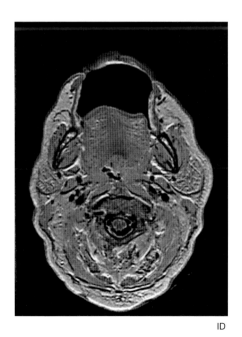

ID

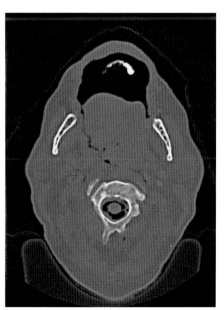

CT

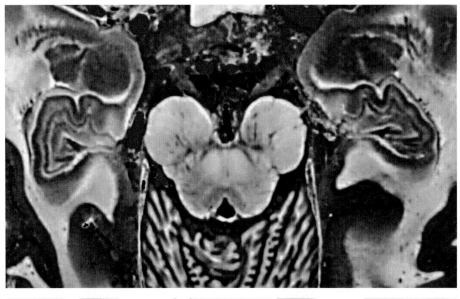

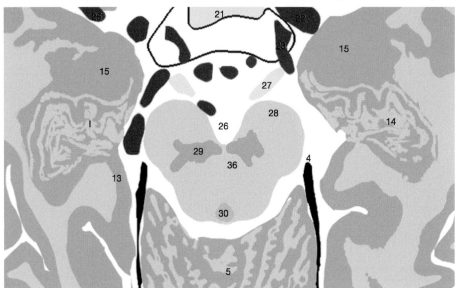

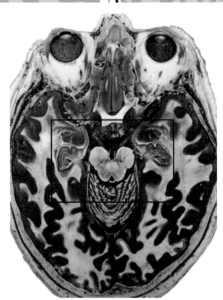

5 – Cerebellum
13 – Parahippocampal gyrus
14 – Hippocampus
15 – Amygdaloid body
21 – Optic chiasm
22 – Internal carotid artery
23 – Posterior communicating artery
25 – Middle cerebral artery
26 – Interpeduncular fossa and cistern
27 – Occulomotor nerve (CN III)
28 – Cerebral peduncle
29 – Substantia nigra
30 – Cerebral aqueduct
36 – Decussation of the superior
     cerebellar peduncles
 I – Dentate gyrus

2
Coronal Sections

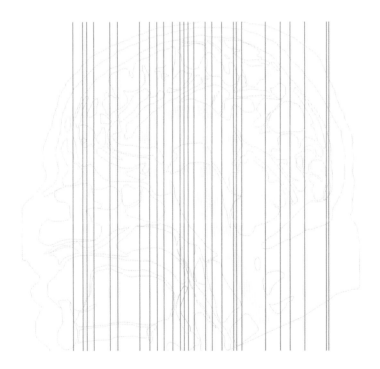

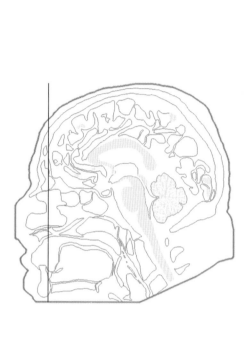

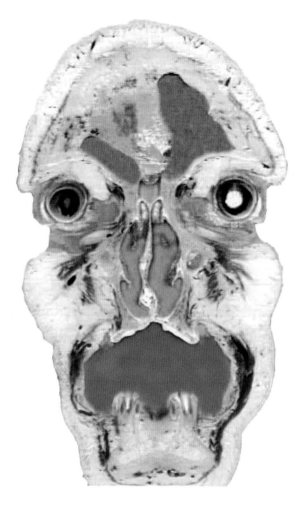

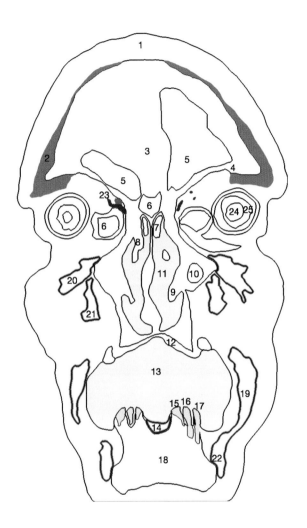

1 – Scalp
2 – Galea aponeurotica
3 – Frontal bone (squama)
4 – Frontal bone (orbital part)
5 – Frontal sinuses
6 – Ethmoidal cells
7 – Superior nasal concha
8 – Middle nasal concha
9 – Inferior nasal concha
10 – Maxillary sinus
11 – Nasal cavity
12 – Hard palate
13 – Oral cavity

14 – Genioglossus muscle
15 – Left lateral inferior incisor tooth
16 – Left inferior canine tooth
17 – Left inferior premolar 1
18 – Mandible
19 – Buccinator muscle
20 – Levator labii superioris muscle
21 – Levator anguli oris muscle
22 – Depressor anguli oris muscle
23 – Angular artery and vein
24 – Lens
25 – Vitreous chamber of the eye

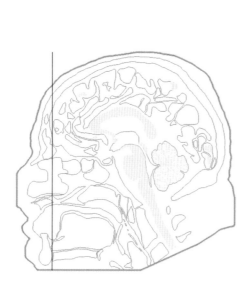

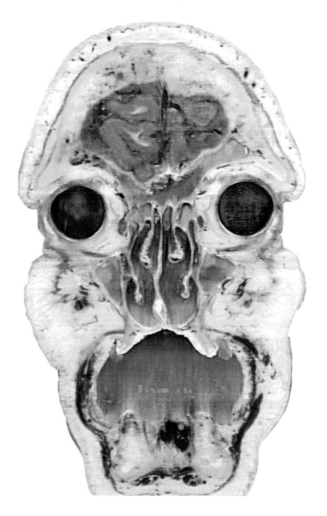

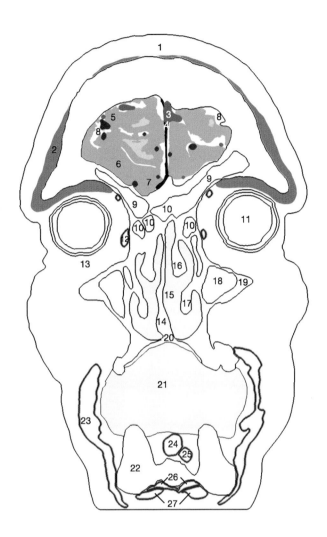

1 – Scalp
2 – Galea aponeurotica
3 – Superior sagittal sinus
4 – Falx cerebri
5 – Middle frontal gyrus
6 – Inferior frontal gyrus
7 – Superior frontal gyrus
8 – Subarachnoid space
     (in the cortical sulci)
9 – Frontal sinus
10 – Ethmoidal cells
11 – Vitreous chamber of the eye
12 – Medial rectus muscle
13 – Inferior oblique muscle

14 – Nasal septum
15 – Nasal cavity
16 – Middle nasal concha
17 – Inferior nasal concha
18 – Maxillary sinus
19 – Maxilla (body)
20 – Hard palate
21 – Oral cavity
22 – Mandible (body)
23 – Buccinator muscle
24 – Genioglossus muscle
25 – Geniolyoid muscle
26 – Mylohyoid muscle
27 – Digastric muscle (anterior belly)

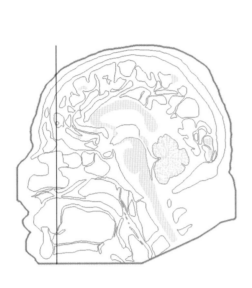

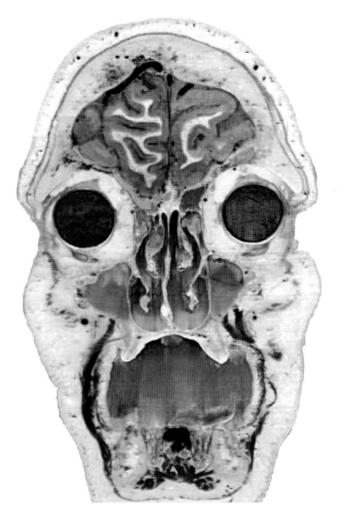

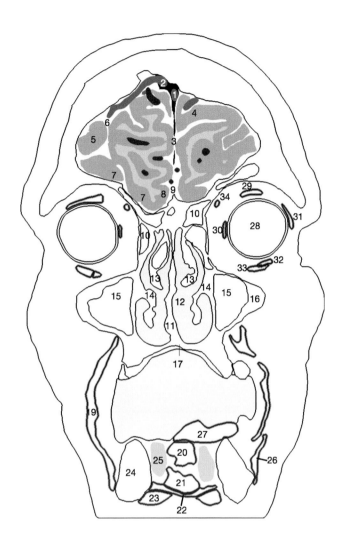

1 – Superior sagittal sinus
2 – Superior cerebral vein, frontal vein)
3 – Falx cerebri
4 – Superior frontal gyrus
5 – Middle frontal gyrus
6 – Superior frontal sulcus
7 – Orbital gyri
8 – Straight gyrus (gyrus rectus)
9 – Crista galli
10 – Ethmoidal cells
11 – Nasal septum
12 – Nasal cavity
13 – Middle nasal concha
14 – Inferior nasal concha
15 – Maxillary sinus
16 – Maxilla (body)
17 – Hard palate

18 – Oral cavity
19 – Buccinator muscle
20 – Genioglossus muscle
21 – Hyoglossus muscle
22 – Mylohyoid muscle
23 – Digastric muscle
24 – Mandible
25 – Sublingual gland
26 – Depressor anguli oris muscle
27 – Tongue
28 – Vitreous chamber of the eye
29 – Superior rectus muscle
30 – Medial rectus muscle
31 – Lateral rectus muscle
32 – Inferior rectus muscle
33 – Inferior oblique muscle
34 – Superior oblique muscle

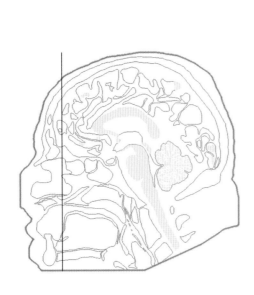

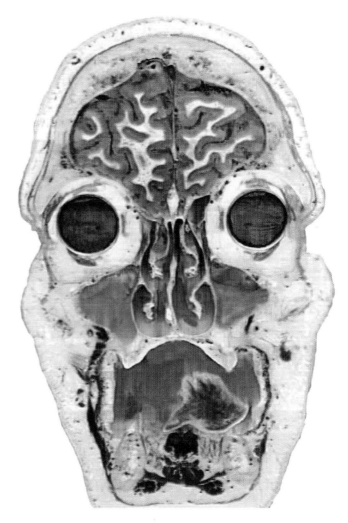

Coronal 300

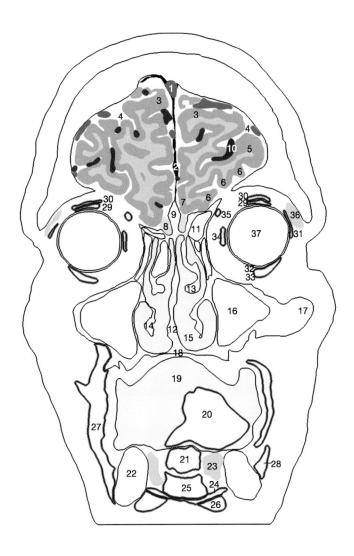

1 – Superior sagittal sinus
2 – Falx cerebri
3 – Superior frontal gyrus
4 – Superior frontal sulcus
5 – Middle frontal gyrus
6 – Orbital gyri
7 – Straight gyrus (gyrus rectus)
8 – Olfactory bulb
9 – Crista galli
10 – Prefrontal artery (branch of middle cerebral artery)
11 – Ethmoidal cells
12 – Nasal septum
13 – Middle nasal concha

14 – Inferior nasal concha
15 – Nasal cavity
16 – Maxillary sinus
17 – Zygomatic process of maxilla
18 – Hard palate
19 – Oral cavity
20 – Tongue
21 – Genioglossus muscle
22 – Mandible
23 – Sublingual gland
24 – Mylohyoid muscle
25 – Geniohyoid muscle

26 – Digastric muscle (anterior belly)
27 – Buccinator muscle
28 – Depressor anguli oris muscle
29 – Superior rectus muscle
30 – Levator palpaebrae superioris muscle
31 – Lateral rectus muscle
32 – Inferior rectus muscle
33 – Inferior oblique muscle
34 – Medial rectus muscle
35 – Superior oblique muscle
36 – Lacrimal gland
37 – Vitreous chamber of the eye

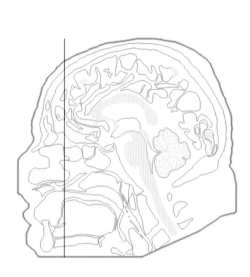

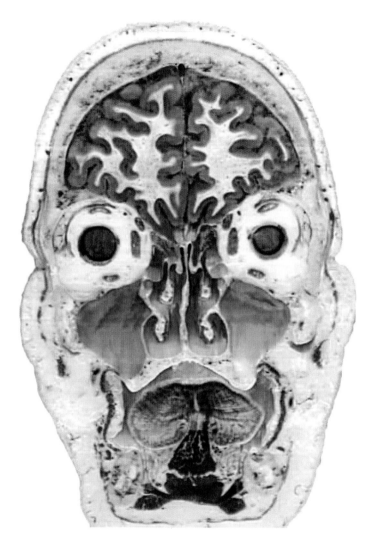

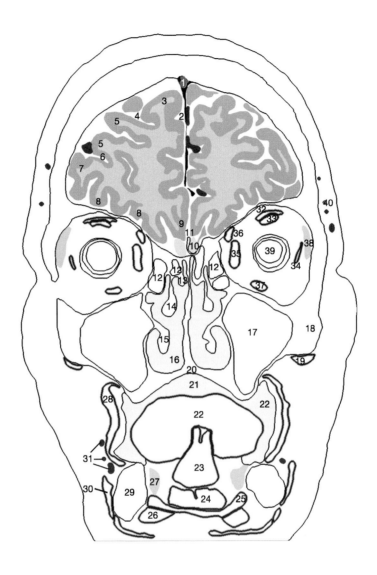

1 – Superior sagittal sinus
2 – Falx cerebri
3 – Superior frontal gyrus
4 – Superior frontal sulcus
5 – Middle frontal gyrus
6 – Inferior frontal sulcus
7 – Inferior frontal gyrus
8 – Orbital gyri
9 – Straight gyrus (gyrus rectus)
10 – Olfactory bulb
11 – Crista galli
12 – Ethmoidal cells
13 – Superior nasal concha
14 – Middle nasal concha
15 – Inferior nasal concha

16 – Nasal cavity
17 – Maxillary sinus
18 – Zygomatic arch
19 – Masetter muscle
(insertion on zygomatic arch)
20 – Hard palate
21 – Oral cavity
22 – Tongue
23 – Genioglossus muscle
24 – Geniohyoid muscle
25 – Mylohyoid muscle
26 – Digastric muscle
(anterior belly)
27 – Submandibular gland
28 – Buccinator muscle

29 – Mandible (body)
30 – Platysma muscle
31 – Facial artery
32 – Levator palpaebrae
superioris muscle
33 – Superior rectus muscle
34 – Lateral rectus muscle
35 – Medial rectus muscle
36 – Superior oblique muscle
37 – Inferior rectus muscle
38 – Lacrimal gland
39 – Vitreous chamber
of the eye
40 – Superficial temporal
artery

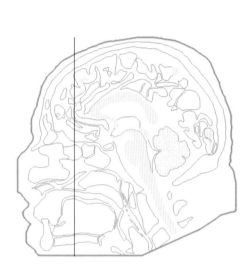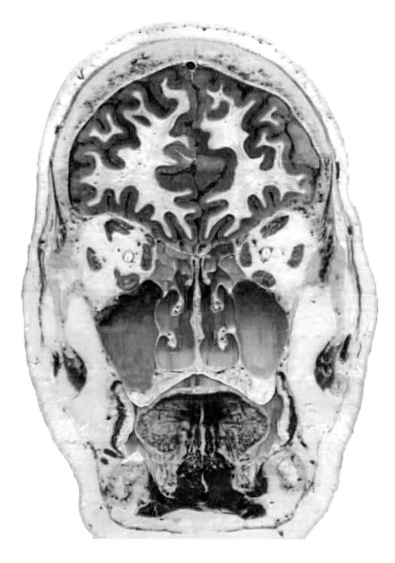

Coronal   400

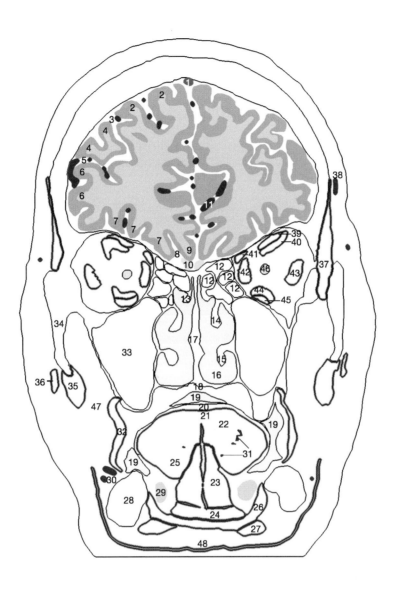

1 – Superior sagittal sinus
2 – Superior frontal gyrus
3 – Superior frontal sulcus
4 – Middle frontal gyrus
5 – Inferior frontal sulcus
6 – Inferior frontal gyrus
7 – Orbital gyri
8 – Olfactory sulcus
9 – Straight gyrus (gyrus rectus)
10 – Olfactory tract
11 – Anteromedial frontal branch
    of pericallosal artery
12 – Ethmoidal cells
13 – Superior nasal concha
14 – Middle nasal concha
15 – Inferior nasal concha
16 – Nasal cavity
17 – Nasal septum

18 – Hard palate
19 – Oral cavity
20 – Tongue mucosa
21 – Superior longitudinal muscle of the
    tongue
22 – Vertical and transverse muscles
    of the tongue
23 – Genioglossus muscle
24 – Geniohyoid muscle
25 – Inferior longitudinal muscle of the tongue
26 – Mylohyoid muscle
27 – Digastric muscle (anterior belly)
28 – Mandible (body)
29 – Sublingual gland
30 – Facial artery
31 – Lingual artery
32 – Buccinator muscle
33 – Maxillary sinus

34 – Zygomatic arch
35 – Massetter muscle (insertion on
    the zygomatic arch)
36 – Zygomatic major muscle
37 – Temporalis muscle
38 – Superficial temporal artery
39 – Levator palpaebrae superioris muscle
40 – Superior rectus muscle
41 – Superior oblique muscle
42 – Medial rectus muscle
43 – Lateral rectus muscle
44 – Inferior rectus muscle
45 – Inferior oblique muscle
46 – Optic nerve (CN II)
47 – Buccal fat body (Bichat's fat pad)
48 – Platysma muscle

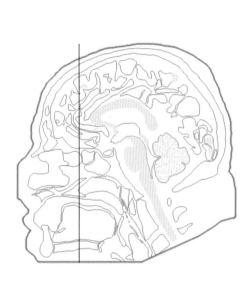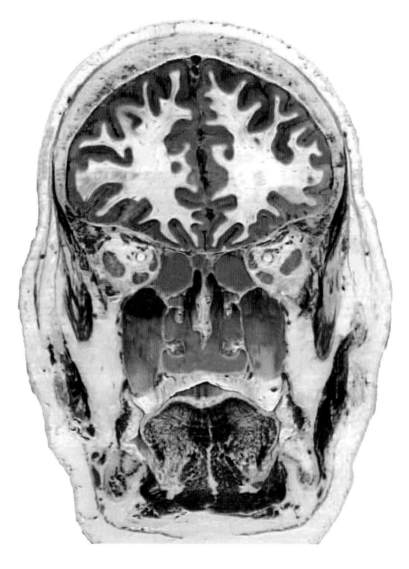

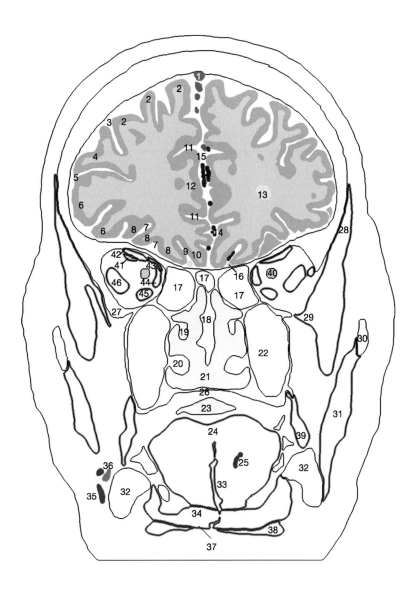

1 – Superior sagittal sinus
2 – Superior frontal gyrus
3 – Superior frontal sulcus
4 – Middle frontal gyrus
5 – Inferior frontal sulcus
6 – Inferior frontal gyrus
7 – Orbital sulci
8 – Orbital gyri
9 – Olfactory sulcus
10 – Straight gyrus (gyrus rectus)
11 – Cingulate sulcus
12 – Cingulate gyrus
13 – Radiation of corpus callosum
14 – Anterior cerebral artery
15 – Anterior cerebral vein
16 – Olfactory tract

17 – Ethmoidal cells
18 – Nasal septum
19 – Middle nasal chonca
20 – Inferior nasal concha
21 – Nasal cavity
22 – Maxillary sinus
23 – Oral cavity
24 – Tongue
25 – Branch of lingual artery
26 – Hard palate
27 – Maxilla (body)
28 – Temporalis muscle
29 – Lateral pterygoid muscle
30 – Mandible (head)
31 – Masseter muscle
32 – Mandible (body)

33 – Genioglossus muscle
34 – Geniohyoid muscle
35 – Facial artery
36 – Facial vein
37 – Mylohyoid muscle
38 – Digastric muscle (anterior belly)
39 – Buccinator muscle
40 – Optic nerve (CN II)
41 – Superior rectus muscle
42 – Levator palpaebrae superioris muscle
43 – Superior oblique muscle
44 – Medial rectus muscle
45 – Inferior rectus muscle
46 – Lateral rectus muscle

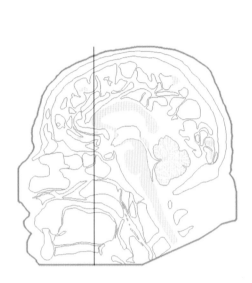

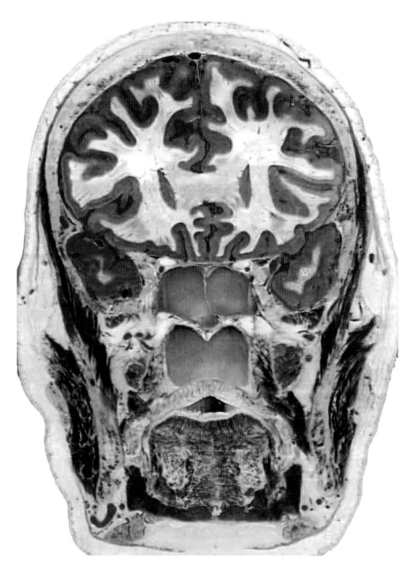

Coronal 530

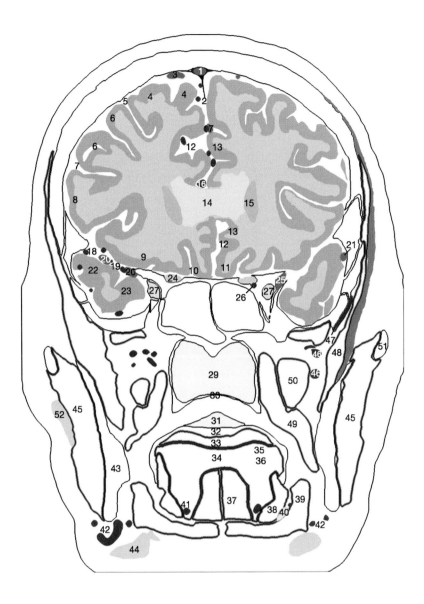

1 – Superior sagittal sinus
2 – Falx cerebri
3 – Superior cerebral vein
4 – Superior frontal gyrus
5 – Superior frontal sulcus
6 – Middle frontal gyrus
7 – Inferior frontal sulcus
8 – Inferior frontal gyrus
9 – Orbital gyri
10 – Olfactory sulcus
11 – Straight gyrus (gyrus rectus)
12 – Cingulate sulcus
13 – Cingulate gyrus
14 – Corpus callosum
15 – Lateral ventricle (anterior horn)
16 – Pericallosal artery
17 – Callosomarginal artery and vein
18 – Lateral sulcus (Sylvius)
19 – Middle cerebral artery

20 – Deep middle cerebral vein
21 – Superficial middle cerebral vein
22 – Superior temporal gyrus
23 – Middle temporal gyrus
24 – Optic nerve (CN II)
25 – Superior ophthalmic vein
26 – Ophthalmic artery
27 – Oculomotor (CN III), Trochlear (CN IV) and Ophthalmic (CN V1), nerves entering the orbit through the superior orbital fissure
28 – Sphenoid sinus
29 – Nasal cavity
30 – Hard palate
31 – Oral cavity
32 – Mucosa of the tongue
33 – Superior longitudinal muscle of the tongue
34 – Vertical and transverse muscles of the tongue

35 – Styloglossus muscle
36 – Inferior longitudinal muscle of the tongue
37 – Genioglossus muscle
38 – Hyoglossus muscle
39 – Mylohyoid muscle
40 – Hypoglossal nerve (CN XII)
41 – Lingual artery
42 – Facial artery
43 – Mandible
44 – Submandibular gland
45 – Masseter muscle
46 – Maxillary artery
47 – Deep temporal artery
48 – Temporalis muscle and fascia
49 – Medial pterygoid muscle
50 – Lateral pterygoid muscle
51 – Zygomatic arch
52 – Parotid gland

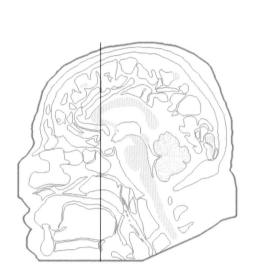

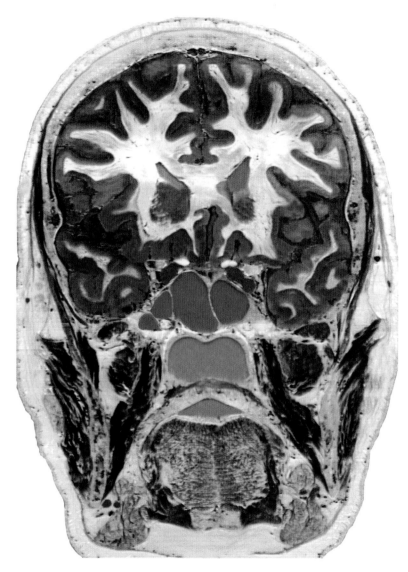

Coronal   570

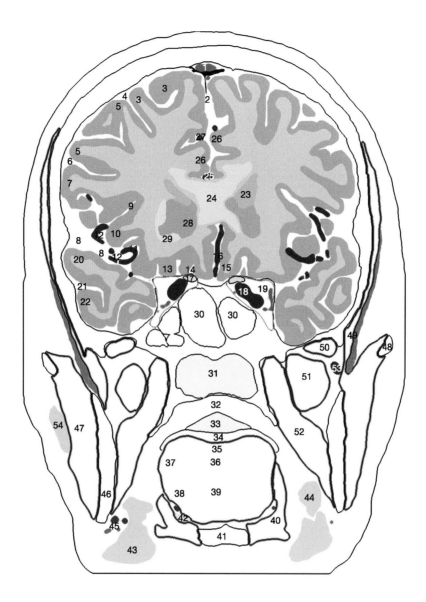

1 – Superior sagittal sinus
2 – Falx cerebri
3 – Superior frontal gyrus
4 – Superior frontal sulcus
5 – Middle frontal gyrus
6 – Inferior frontal sulcus
7 – Inferior frontal gyrus
8 – Lateral sulcus (Sylvius)
9 – Circular insular sulcus
10 – Short insular gyri
11 – Central insular sulcus
12 – Middle cerebral artery
13 – Orbital gyri
14 – Olfactory sulcus
15 – Straight gyrus (gyrus rectus)
16 – Anterior cerebral artery
17 – Optic nerve (CN II)
18 – Internal carotid artery
19 – Cavernous sinus

20 – Superior temporal gyrus
21 – Superior temporal sulcus
22 – Middle temporal gyrus
23 – Lateral ventricle (anterior horn)
24 – Corpus callosum (rostrum)
25 – Pericallosal arteries
26 – Cingulate gyrus
27 – Callosomarginal artery
28 – Head of caudate nucleus
29 – Internal capsule (anterior limb)
30 – Sphenoid sinus
31 – Nasal cavity
32 – Soft palate
33 – Oral cavity
34 – Mucosa of the tongue
35 – Superior longitudinal muscle
     of the tongue
36 – Vertical and transverse muscles
     of the tongue

37 – Styloglossus muscle
38 – Inferior longitudinal muscle of the tongue
39 – Genioglossus muscle
40 – Hyoglossus muscle
41 – Hyoid bone
42 – Hypoglossal nerve (CN XII)
43 – Submandibular gland
44 – Sublingual gland
45 – Facial artery and vein
46 – Mandible (ramus)
47 – Masseter muscle
48 – Zygomatic arch
49 – Temporalis muscle and fascia
50 – Lateral pterygoid muscle (upper head)
51 – Lateral pterygoid muscle (lower head)
52 – Medial pterygoid muscle
53 – Maxillary artery
54 – Parotid gland

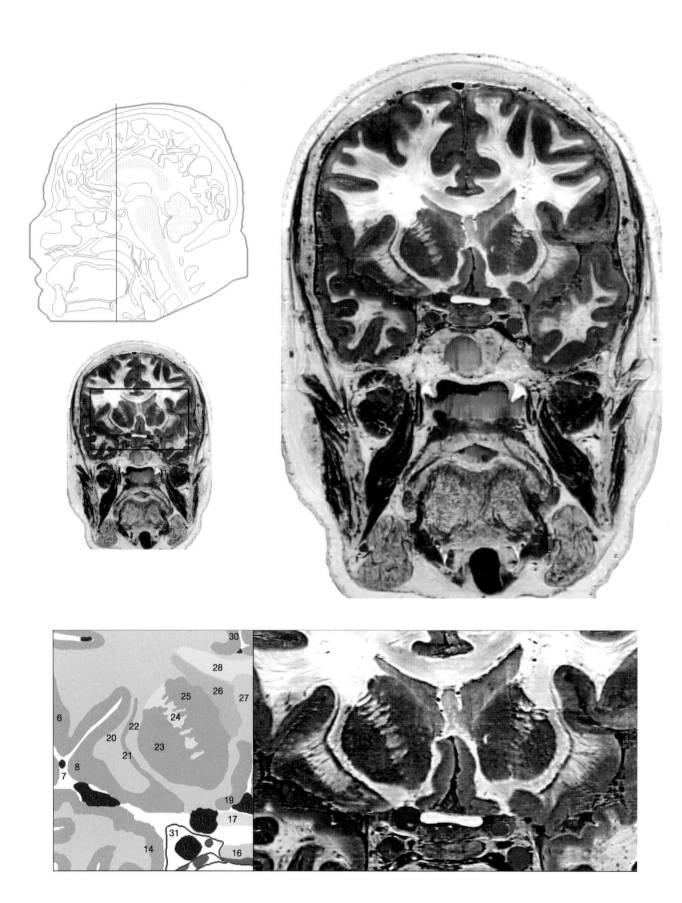

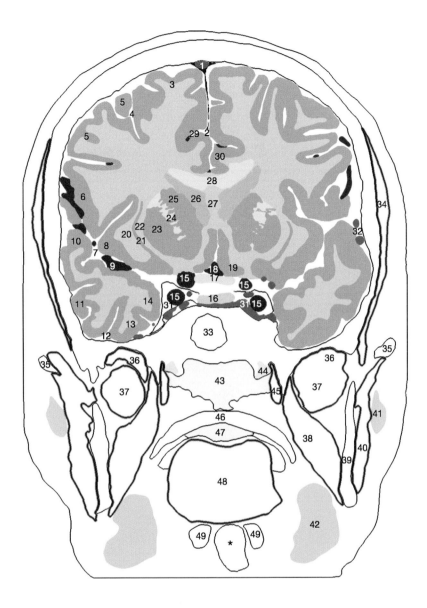

1 – Superior sagittal sinus
2 – Falx cerebri
3 – Superior frontal gyrus
4 – Superior frontal sulcus
5 – Middle frontal gyrus
6 – Inferior frontal gyrus
7 – Lateral sulcus (Sylvius)
8 – Insula
9 – Middle cerebral artery
10 – Superior temporal gyrus
11 – Middle temporal gyrus
12 – Inferior temporal sulcus
13 – Inferior temporal gyrus
14 – Parahippocampal gyrus
15 – Internal carotid artery
16 – Pituitary gland
17 – Optic chiasm

18 – Anterior cerebral artery
19 – Straight gyrus (gyrus rectus)
20 – Extreme capsule
21 – Claustrum
22 – External capsule
23 – Putamen
24 – Internal capsule (anterior limb)
25 – Head of caudate nucleus
26 – Lateral ventricle (anterior horn)
27 – Pellucid septum
28 – Corpus callosum
29 – Cingulate sulcus
30 – Cingulate girus
31 – Cavernous sinus
32 – Superficial middle cerebral vein
33 – Sphenoid sinus
34 – Temporalis muscle and fascia

35 – Zygomatic arch
36 – Lateral pterygoid muscle (upper head)
37 – Lateral pterygoid muscle (lower head)
38 – Medial pterygoid muscle
39 – Mandible
40 – Masseter muscle
41 – Parotid gland
42 – Submandibular gland
43 – Rhinopharynx
44 – Pharyngotympanic (auditory) tube (Eustachio)
45 – Tensor veli palatini muscle
46 – Soft palate
47 – Oral cavity
48 – Tongue
49 – Hyoid bone
 * – Cyst of the thyreoglossal duct

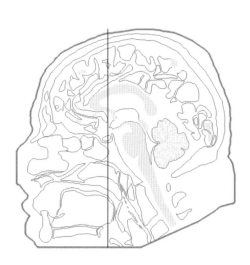

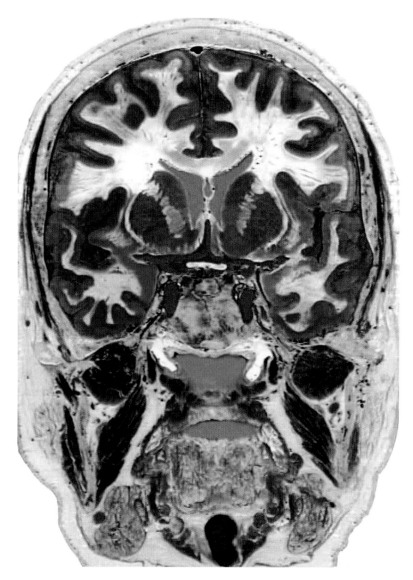

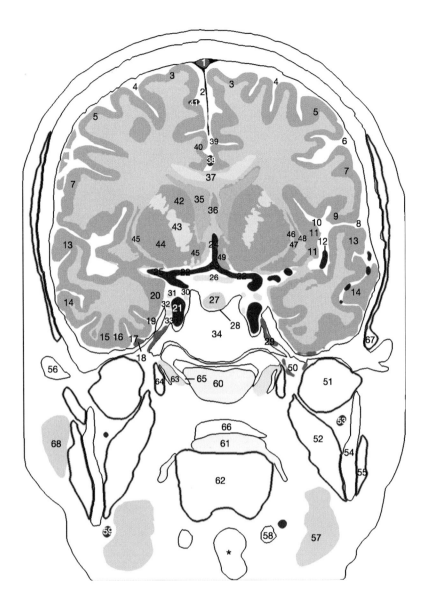

1 – Superior sagittal sinus
2 – Falx cerebri
3 – Superior frontal gyrus
4 – Superior frontal sulcus
5 – Middle frontal gyrus
6 – Inferior frontal sulcus
7 – Inferior frontal gyrus
8 – Lateral sulcus (Sylvius)
9 – Inferior frontal gyrus, opercular part
10 – Circular insular sulcus
11 – Short insular gyri
12 – Middle cerebral artery
13 – Superior temporal gyrus
14 – Middle temporal gyrus
15 – Inferior temporal sulcus
16 – Lateral occipitotemporal gyrus
17 – Collateral sulcus
18 – Uncal vein
19 – Rhinal sulcus
20 – Parahippocampal gyrus
21 – Internal carotid artery
22 – Anterior cerebral artery, A1 segment
23 – Anterior communicating artery
24 – Anterior cerebral artery, A2 segment

25 – Middle cerebral artery, M1 segment
26 – Optic chiasm
27 – Pituitary gland
28 – Sella turcica
29 – Cavernous sinus
30 – Oculomotor nerve (CN III)
31 – Trochlear nerve (CN IV)
32 – Abducent nerve (CN VI)
33 – Ophthalmic nerve (CN V1)
34 – Sphenoid bone (body)
35 – Lateral ventricle (anterior horn)
36 – Pellucid septum with cavum septi pellucidi
37 – Corpus callosum
38 – Pericallosal artery
39 – Cingulate sulcus
40 – Cingulate gyrus
41 – Callosomarginal artery
42 – Head of caudate nucleus
43 – Internal capsule (anterior limb)
44 – Putamen
45 – Nucleus accumbens
46 – External capsule
47 – Claustrum

48 – Extreme capsule
49 – Straight gyrus (gyrus rectus)
50 – Pterygoid venous plexus
51 – Lateral pterygoid muscle
52 – Medial pterygoid muscle
53 – Maxilary artery
54 – Mandible
55 – Masseter muscle
56 – Zygomatic arch
57 – Submandibular gland
58 – Hyoid bone
59 – Facial artery
60 – Rhinopharinx
61 – Oral cavity
62 – Tongue
63 – Pharyngotympanic (auditory) tube (Eustachio)
64 – Tensor veli palatini muscle
65 – Pterygoid process (hamulus)
66 – Soft palate
67 – Temporalis muscle and fascia
68 – Parotid gland
 * – Cyst of the thyreoglossal duct

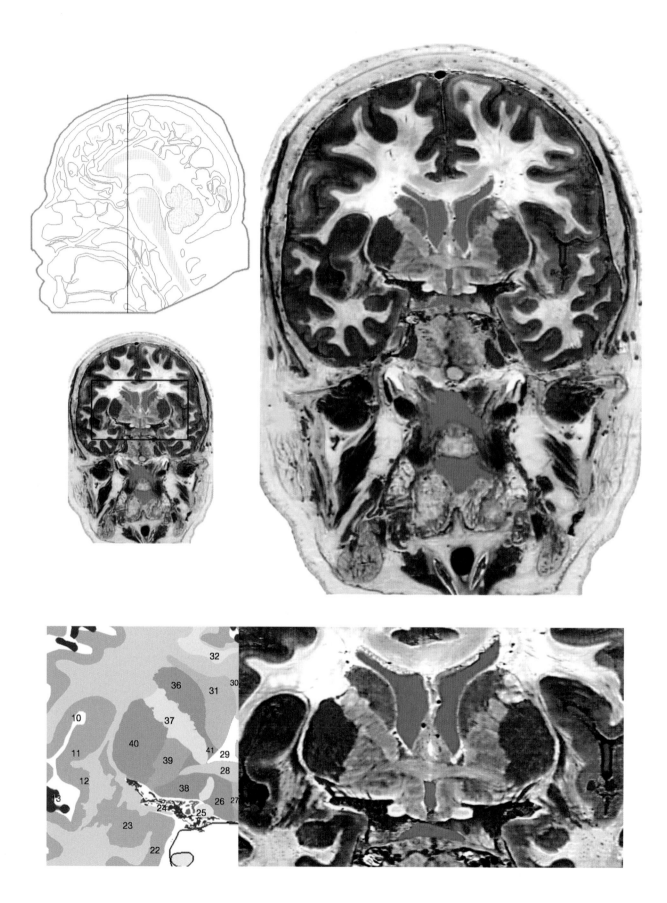

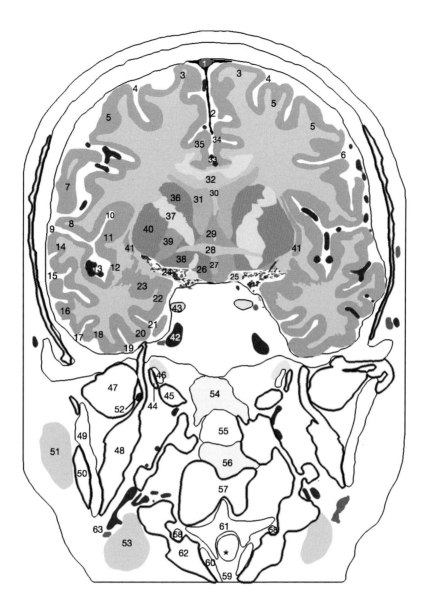

1 – Superior sagittal sinus
2 – Falx cerebri
3 – Superior frontal gyrus
4 – Superior frontal sulcus
5 – Middle frontal gyrus
6 – Precentral sulcus
7 – Precentral gyrus (motor strip)
8 – Inferior frontal gyrus, opercular part
9 – Lateral sulcus (Sylvius)
10 – Circular insular sulcus
11 – Short insular gyri
12 – Long insular gyrus
13 – Middle cerebral artery
14 – Superior temporal gyrus
15 – Superior temporal sulcus
16 – Middle temporal gyrus
17 – Inferior temporal sulcus
18 – Inferior temporal gyrus
19 – Collateral sulcus
20 – Lateral occipitotemporal gyrus
21 – Rhinal sulcus
22 – Parahippocampal gyrus
23 – Amygdaloid body

24 – Central anterolateral arteries branching from the middle cerebral artery and penetrating through the substantia perforanta anterior
25 – Optic tract
26 – Hypothalamus
27 – Optic recess of the third ventricle
28 – Anterior commissure
29 – Fornix (body)
30 – Pellucid septum
31 – Lateral ventricle
32 – Corpus callosum
33 – Pericallosal artery
34 – Cingulate sulcus
35 – Cingulate gyrus
36 – Head of caudate nucleus
37 – Internal capsule (anterior limb)
38 – Globus pallidus pars interna (GPi)
39 – Globus pallidus pars externa (GPe)
40 – Putamen
41 – Claustrum
42 – Internal carotid artery
43 – Oculomotor nerve (CN III)

44 – Tensor veli palatini muscle
45 – Levator veli palatini muscle
46 – Pharyngotympanic (auditory) tube (Eustachio)
47 – Lateral pterygoid muscle
48 – Medial pterygoid muscle
49 – Mandible (ramus)
50 – Masseter muscle
51 – Parotid gland
52 – Maxillary artery
53 – Submandibular gland
54 – Rhinopharinx
55 – Soft palate
56 – Oropharynx
57 – Tongue
58 – Hyoid bone
59 – Larynx
60 – Thyroid cartilage
61 – Thyrohyoid membrane
62 – Thyrohyoid muscle
63 – Facial artery and vein
* – Cyst of the thyreoglossal duct

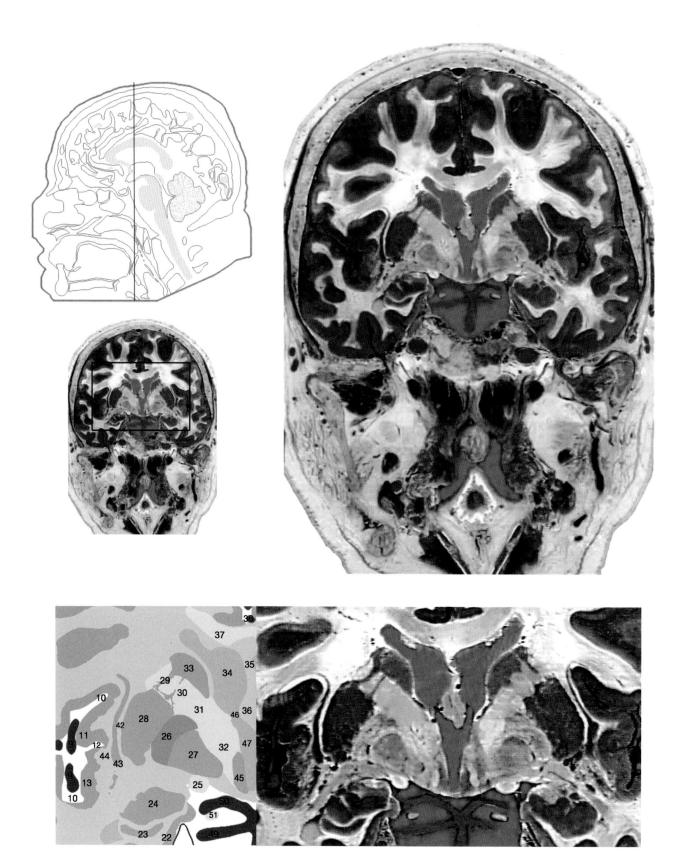

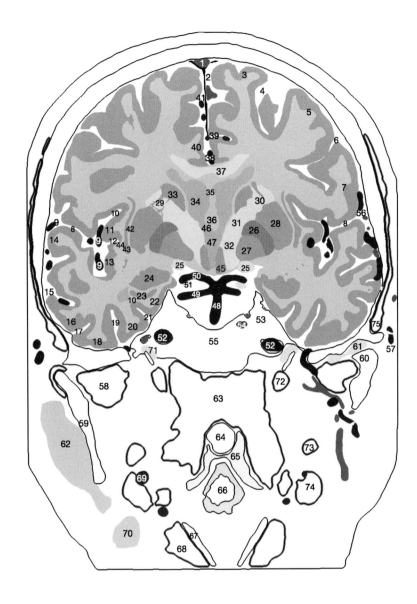

1 – Superior sagittal sinus
2 – Falx cerebri
3 – Superior frontal gyrus
4 – Superior frontal sulcus
5 – Middle frontal gyrus
6 – Precentral sulcus
7 – Precentral gyrus
8 – Lateral sulcus (Sylvius)
9 – Middle cerebral artery
10 – Circular insular sulcus
11 – Short insular gyri
12 – Central insular sulcus
13 – Long insular gyrus
14 – Superior temporal gyrus
15 – Superior temporal sulcus
16 – Middle temporal gyrus
17 – Inferior temporal sulcus
18 – Inferior temporal gyrus
19 – Collateral sulcus
20 – Lateral occipitotemporal gyrus
21 – Rhinal sulcus
22 – Parahippocampal gyrus
23 – Amygdaloid body
24 – Hippocampus
25 – Optic tract

26 – Globus pallidus pars externa (GPe)
27 – Globus pallidus pars interna (GPi)
28 – Putamen
29 – Caudato-lenticular gray matter bridges
30 – Internal capsule (anterior limb)
31 – Internal capsule (genu)
32 – Internal capsule (posterior limb)
33 – Head of caudate nucleus
34 – Lateral ventricle
35 – Pellucid septum
36 – Fornix body
37 – Corpus callosum
38 – Pericallosal artery
39 – Cingulate sulcus
40 – Cingulate gyrus
41 – Callosomarginal artery
42 – External capsule
43 – Claustrum
44 – Extreme capsule
45 – Hypothalamus
46 – Interventricular foramen (Monro)
47 – Third ventricle
48 – Basilar artery
49 – Superior cerebellar artery
50 – Posterior cerebral artery

51 – Oculomotor nerve (CN III)
52 – Internal carotid artery
53 – Cavernous sinus
54 – Basilar venous plexus
55 – Basilar process of the sphenoid
56 – Superficial middle cerebral vein
57 – Superficial temporal artery
58 – Lateral pterygoid muscle
59 – Mandible (ramus)
60 – Head of mandible
61 – Articular disc, temporo-mandibular joint
62 – Parotid gland
63 – Soft palate
64 – Uvula
65 – Oropharynx
66 – Epiglottis
67 – Thyroid cartilage
68 – Sternothyroid muscle
69 – Lingual artery
70 – Submanidibular gland
71 – Pharyngotympanic (auditory) tube (Eustachio)
72 – Levator veli palatini muscle
73 – Stylohyoid muscle
74 – Styloglossus muscle
75 – Temporalis muscle and fascia

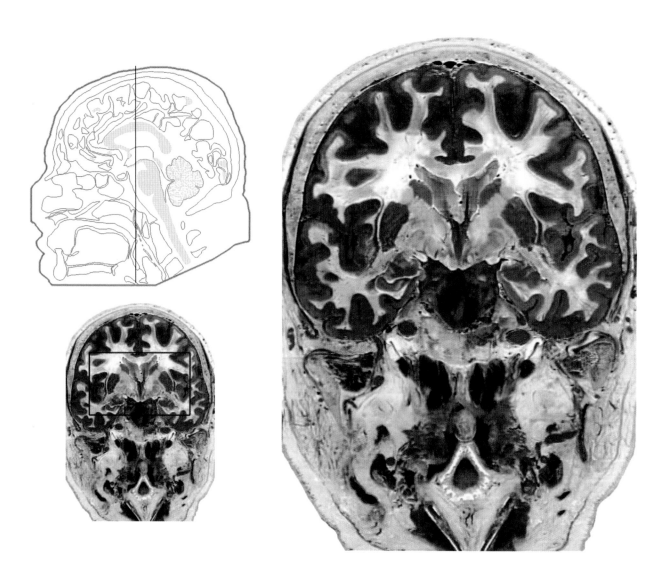

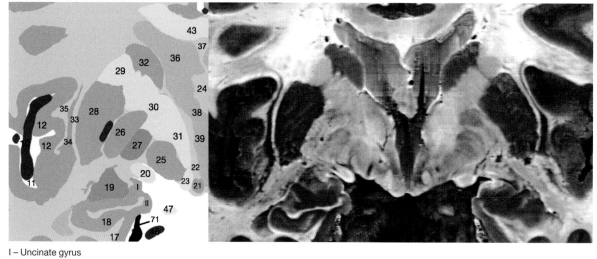

I – Uncinate gyrus
II – Ambiens gyrus

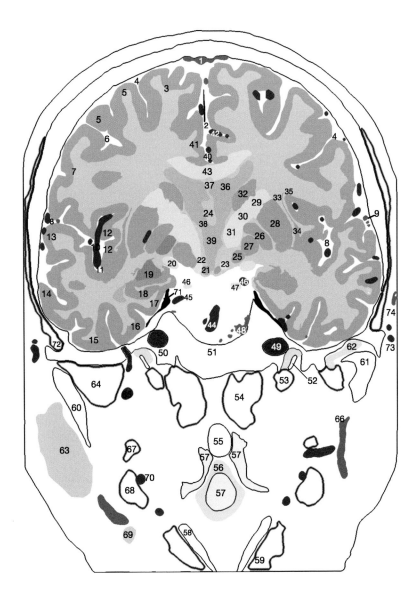

1 – Superior sagittal sinus
2 – Falx cerebri
3 – Superior frontal gyrus
4 – Superior frontal sulcus
5 – Middle frontal gyrus
6 – Precentral sulcus
7 – Precentral gyrus
8 – Lateral sulcus (Sylvius)
9 – Superficial middle temporal vein
10 – Middle cerebral artery
11 – Circular insular sulcus
12 – Long insular gyrus
13 – Superior temporal gyrus
14 – Middle temporal gyrus
15 – Inferior temporal gyrus
16 – Lateral occipitotemporal gyrus
17 – Parahippocampal gyrus
18 – Hippocampus
19 – Amygdaloid body
20 – Optic tract
21 – Mamillary body
22 – Hypothalamus
23 – Mamillo-thalamic tract
24 – Fornix (body)
25 – Subthalamic nucleus

26 – Globus pallidus pars externa (GPe)
27 – Globus pallidus pars interna (GPi)
28 – Putamen
29 – Internal capsule (anterior limb)
30 – Internal capsule (genu)
31 – Internal capsule (posterior limb)
32 – Head of caudate nucleus
33 – External capsule
34 – Claustrum
35 – Extreme capsule
36 – Lateral ventricle
37 – Pellucid septum
38 – Interventricular foramen (Monro)
39 – Third ventricle
40 – Pericallosal artery
41 – Cingulate gyrus
42 – Cingulate sulcus, callosomarginal artery
43 – Corpus callosum
44 – Basilar artery
45 – Anterior inferior cerebellar artery (AICA)
46 – Posterior cerebral artery
47 – Oculomotor nerve (CN III)
48 – Basilar venous plexus
49 – Internal carotid artery in the carotid canal
50 – Petrous bone

51 – Basilar process of the sphenoid bone
52 – Pharyngotympanic (auditory) tube (Eustachio)
53 – Levator veli palatini muscle
54 – Soft palate
55 – Uvula
56 – Epiglottis
57 – Oropharynx
58 – Thyroid cartilage
59 – Sternohyoid muscle
60 – Mandible (ramus)
61 – Head of mandible
62 – Temporo-mandibular joint, articular disc
63 – Parotid gland
64 – Lateral pterygoid muscle
65 – Maxillary artery
66 – Retromandibular vein
67 – Stylohyoid muscle
68 – Styloglossus muscle
69 – Submandibular gland
70 – Lingual artery
71 – Tentorium cerebelli
72 – Temporalis muscle and fascia
73 – Superficial temporal artery
74 – Superficial temporal vein

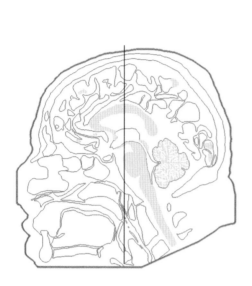

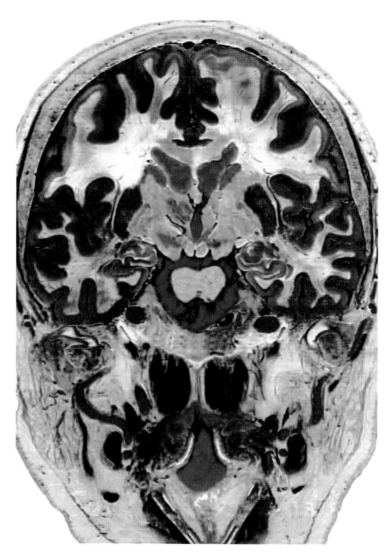

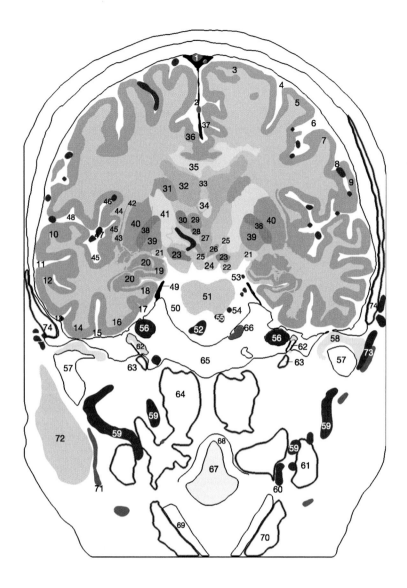

1 – Superior sagittal sinus
2 – Falx cerebri
3 – Superior frontal gyrus
4 – Superior frontal sulcus
5 – Middle frontal gyrus
6 – Precentral sulcus
7 – Precentral gyrus
8 – Central sulcus
9 – Postcentral gyrus
10 – Superior temporal gyrus
11 – Superior temporal sulcus
12 – Middle temporal gyrus
13 – Inferior temporal sulcus
14 – Inferior temporal gyrus
15 – Occipitotemporal sulcus
16 – Lateral occipitotemporal gyrus
17 – Rhinal sulcus
18 – Parahippocampal gyrus
19 – Uncinate gyrus
20 – Hippocampus
21 – Optic tract
22 – Cerebral peduncle
23 – Substantia nigra
24 – Mamillary body
25 – Mamillo-thalamic tract
26 – Subthalamic nucleus

27 – Third ventricle
28 – Medial thalamic nucleus
29 – Anterior thalamic nucleus
30 – Ventral lateral thalamic nucleus
31 – Head of caudate nucleus
32 – Lateral ventricle
33 – Pellucid septum
34 – Fornix body
35 – Corpus callosum
36 – Cingulate gyrus
37 – Cingulate sulcus
38 – Globus pallidus pars externa (GPe)
39 – Globus pallidus pars interna (GPi)
40 – Putamen
41 – Internal capsule (posterior limb)
42 – External capsule
43 – Claustrum
44 – Extreme capsule
45 – Insula
46 – Circular insular sulcus
47 – Middle cerebral artery
48 – Lateral sulcus (Sylvius)
49 – Tentorium cerebelli
50 – Pontocerebellar cistern
51 – Pons
52 – Basilar artery

53 – Posterior cerebral artery
54 – Lateral pontine arteries
55 – Medial pontine arteries
56 – Internal carotid artery passing through
   the carotid canal
57 – Head of mandible
58 – Tempro-mandibular joint, articular disc
59 – Maxillary artery
60 – Lingual artery
61 – Styloglossus muscle
62 – Pharyngotympanic (auditory) tube
   (Eustachio)
63 – Levator veli palatini muscle
64 – Longus capitis muscle
65 – Basilar process of the occipital bone
66 – Basilar venous plexus
67 – Oropharynx
68 – Epiglottis
69 – Thyroid cartilage
70 – Sternothyroid muscle
71 – Retromandibular vein
72 – Parotid gland
73 – Superficial temporal artery
74 – Temporalis muscle and fascia

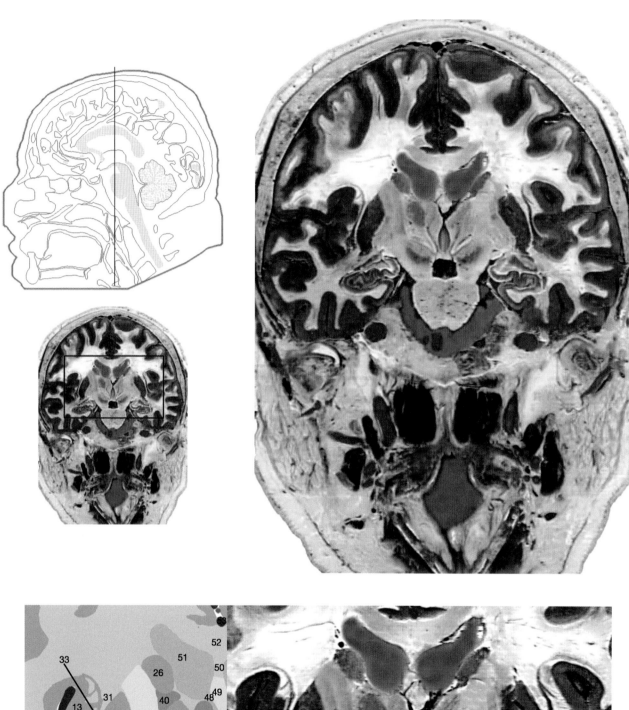

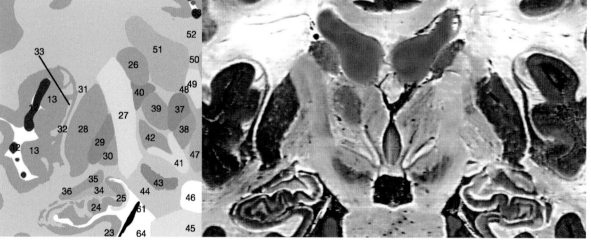

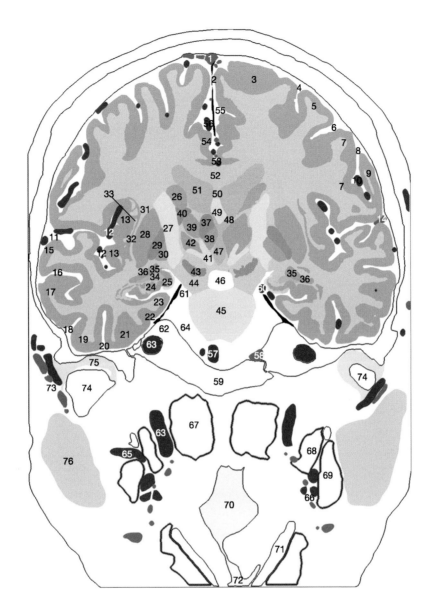

1 – Superior sagittal sinus
2 – Falx cerebri
3 – Superior frontal gyrus
4 – Superior frontal sulcus
5 – Middle frontal gyrus
6 – Precentral sulcus
7 – Precentral gyrus
8 – Central sulcus
9 – Postcentral gyrus
10 – Artery of the central sulcus (branch of middle cerebral artery)
11 – Lateral sulcus (Sylvius)
12 – Middle cerebral artery
13 – Long insular gyrus
14 – Superficial middle cerebral vein
15 – Superior temporal gyrus
16 – Superior temporal sulcus
17 – Middle temporal gyrus
18 – Inferior temporal sulcus
19 – Inferior temporal gyrus

20 – Occipitotemporal sulcus
21 – Lateral occipitotemporal gyrus
22 – Rhinal sulcus
23 – Parahippocampal gyrus
24 – Hippocampus
25 – Uncinate gyrus
26 – Head of caudate nucleus
27 – Internal capsule (posterior limb)
28 – Putamen
29 – Globus pallidus (pars) externa (GPe)
30 – Globus pallidus (pars) interna (GPi)
31 – External capsule
32 – Claustrum
33 – Extreme capsule
34 – Temporal horn of the lateral ventricle
35 – Medial geniculate body
36 – Lateral geniculate body
37 – Anterior thalamic nucleus
38 – Medial thalamic nucleus
39 – Ventral lateral nucleus of thalamus

40 – Reticular nucleus of thalamus
41 – Mamillo-thalamic tract
42 – Ventral posterolateral nucleus of thalamus (VPL)
43 – Substantia nigra
44 – Cerebral peduncle
45 – Pons
46 – Interpeduncular fossa and cistern
47 – Third ventricle
48 – Interventricular foramen (Monro)
49 – Fornix body
50 – Pellucid septum
51 – Lateral ventricle (frontal horn)
52 – Corpus callosum
53 – Pericallosal artery
54 – Cingulate gyrus
55 – Cingulate sulcus
56 – Callosomarginal artery
57 – Basilar artery
58 – Basilar venous plexus

59 – Basilar process of the occipital bone
60 – Anterior choroidal artery
61 – Tentorium
62 – Petrous bone
63 – Internal carotid artery passing through the carotid canal
64 – Pontocerebellar cistern
65 – Maxillary artery
66 – Lingual artery
67 – Longus capitis muscle
68 – Stylohyoid muscle
69 – Styloglossus muscle
70 – Oropharynx
71 – Thyroid cartilage
72 – Larynx
73 – Superficial temporal artery and vein
74 – Head of mandible
75 – Temporomandibular joint, articular disc
76 – Parotid gland

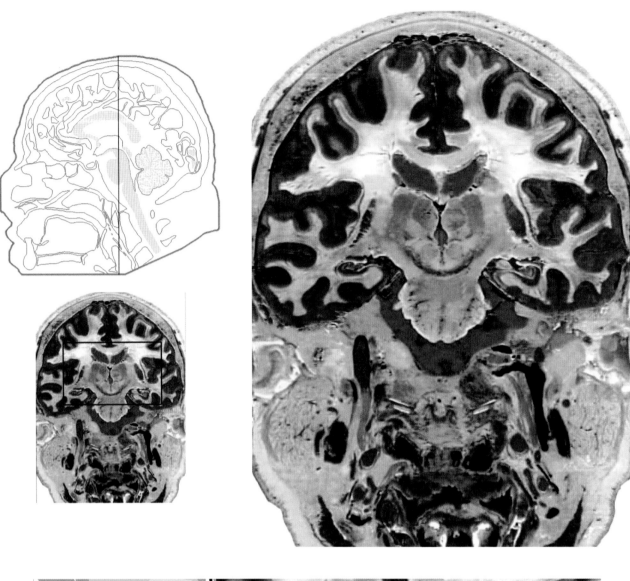

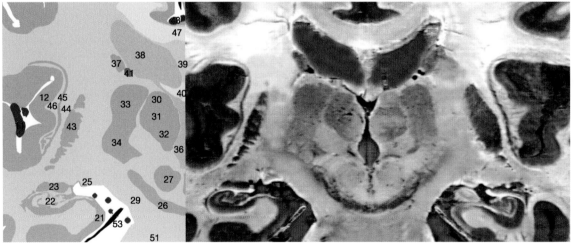

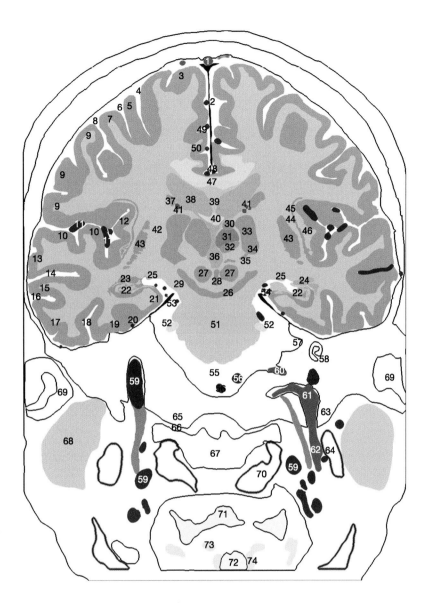

1 – Superior sagittal sinus
2 – Falx cerebri
3 – Superior frontal gyrus
4 – Superior frontal sulcus
5 – Middle frontal gyrus
6 – Precentral sulcus
7 – Precentral gyrus
8 – Central sulcus
9 – Postcentral gyrus
10 – Planum temporale (transverse temporal gyri Heschl)
11 – Middle cerebral artery
12 – Insula
13 – Superior temporal gyrus
14 – Superior temporal sulcus
15 – Middle temporal gyrus
16 – Middle temporal sulcus
17 – Inferior temporal gyrus
18 – Occipitotemporal sulcus
19 – Lateral occipitotemporal gyrus

20 – Rhinal sulcus
21 – Parahippocampal gyrus
22 – Hippocampus
23 – Tail of caudate nucleus
24 – Temporal horn of the lateral ventricle
25 – Medial geniculate body
26 – Substantia nigra
27 – Red nucleus
28 – Decussation of the superior cerebellar peduncles
29 – Cerebral peduncle
30 – Lateral dorsal thalamic nucleus
31 – Medial nucleus of thalamus
32 – Centromedian nucleus of thalamus
33 – Ventral lateral nucleus of thalamus
34 – Ventral posterolateral nucleus of thalamus (VPL)
35 – Subthalamic nucleus

36 – Third ventricle
37 – Head of caudate nucleus
38 – Lateral ventricle (frontal horn)
39 – Pellucid septum
40 – Fornix commissure
41 – Thalamostriate vein
42 – Internal capsule (posterior limb)
43 – Putamen
44 – External capsule
45 – Claustrum
46 – Extreme capsule
47 – Corpus callosum
48 – Pericallosal artery
49 – Cingulate sulcus
50 – Cingulate gyrus
51 – Pons
52 – Trigeminal nerve (CN V)
53 – Tentorium cerebelli
54 – Anterior choroidal artery
55 – Pontocerebellar cistern

56 – Vertebral arteries
57 – Internal acoustic meatus
58 – Internal ear
59 – Internal carotid artery
60 – Inferior petrosal sinus
61 – Bulb of jugular vein
62 – Internal jugular vein
63 – Mastoid process
64 – Digastric muscle (posterior belly)
65 – Occipital condyle
66 – Atlanto-occipital joint
67 – Atlas
68 – Parotid gland
69 – External auditory canal
70 – Rectus capitis muscle
71 – Oropharynx
72 – Larynx
73 – Arytenoid cartilage
74 – Crycoid cartilage

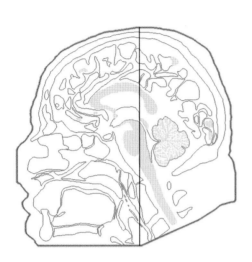

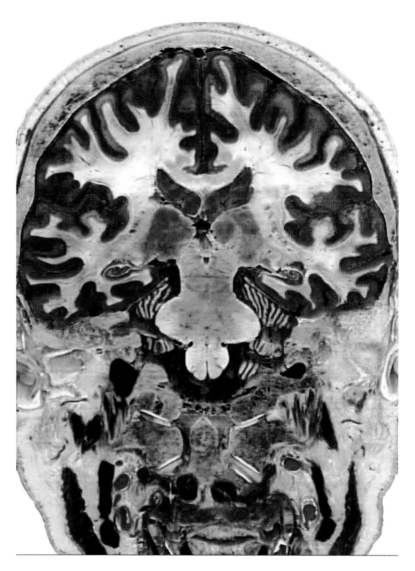

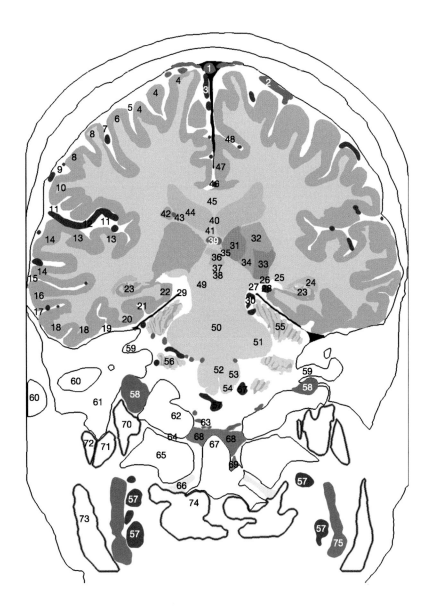

1 – Superior sagittal sinus
2 – Superior cerebral vein, frontal vein
3 – Paracentral artery
4 – Superior frontal gyrus
5 – Precentral sulcus
6 – Precentral gyrus
7 – Central sulcus
8 – Postcentral gyrus
9 – Postcentral sulcus
10 – Supramaginal gyrus
11 – Lateral sulcus (Sylvius)
12 – Middle cerebral artery
13 – Planum temporale (transverse temporal gyri Heschl)
14 – Superior temporal gyrus
15 – Superior temporal sulcus
16 – Middle temporal gyrus
17 – Inferior temporal sulcus
18 – Inferior temporal gyrus
19 – Occipitotemporal sulcus

20 – Lateral occipitotemporal gyrus
21 – Rhinal sulcus
22 – Parahippocampal gyrus
23 – Hippocampus
24 – Temporal horn of the lateral ventricle
25 – Lateral geniculate body
26 – Medial geniculate body
27 – Perimesencephalic cistern
28 – Anterior choroidal artery
29 – Tentorium cerebelli
30 – Superior cerebellar artery
31 – Medial thalamic nucleus
32 – Ventral lateral thalamic nucleus
33 – Ventral posterolateral thalamic nucleus (VPL)
34 – Centromedian thalamic nucleus
35 – Nuclei of habenula
36 – Third ventricle

37 – Posterior commissure
38 – Cerebral aqueduct
39 – Internal cerebral veins
40 – Pellucid septum
41 – Fornix commissure
42 – Caudate nucleus
43 – Thalamostriate vein
44 – Lateral ventricle
45 – Corpus callosum
46 – Pericallosal artery
47 – Cingulate gyrus
48 – Cingulate sulcus
49 – Cerebral peduncle
50 – Pons
51 – Middle cerebellar peduncle
52 – Medulla oblongata
53 – Oliva
54 – Pyramid
55 – Cerebellar hemisphere
56 – Flocculus

57 – Vertebral arteries
58 – Bulb of jugular vein
59 – Internal acoustic meatus
60 – External auditory canal
61 – Mastoid process
62 – Occipital condyle
63 – Basilar venous plexus
64 – Atlanto-occipital joint
65 – Massa lateralis of atlas
66 – Lateral atlanto-axial joint
67 – Dens of axis
68 – Allar ligaments
69 – Transverse ligament of atlas
70 – Rectus capitis lateralis muscle
71 – Digastric muscle (posterior belly)
72 – Stylohyoid muscle
73 – Sternocleidomastoid muscle
74 – Longus colli muscle
75 – Internal jugular vein

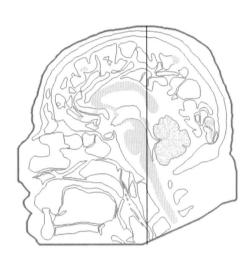

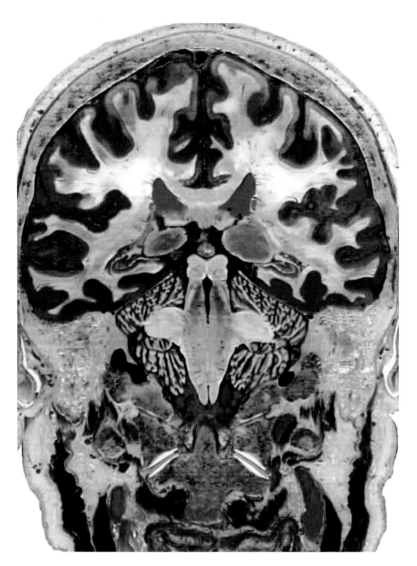

Coronal   900

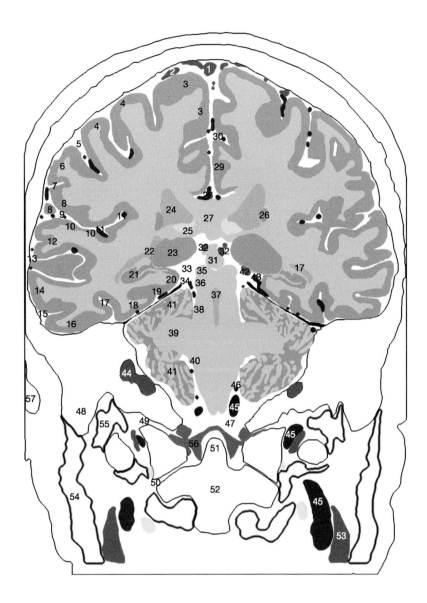

1 – Superior sagittal sinus
2 – Superior cerebral veins, frontal veins
3 – Paracentral lobule
4 – Precentral gyrus
5 – Central sulcus
6 – Postcentral gyrus
7 – Postcentral sulcus
8 – Supramarginal gyrus
9 – Lateral sulcus (Sylvius)
10 – Planum temporale (transverse
      temporal gyri Heschl)
11 – Middle cerebral artery
12 – Superior temporal gyrus
13 – Superior temporal sulcus
14 – Middle temporal gyrus
15 – Inferior temporal sulcus
16 – Inferior temporal gyrus
17 – Occipitotemporal sulcus
18 – Lateral occipitotemporal gyrus
19 – Rhinal sulcus

20 – Parahippocampal gyrus
21 – Hippocampus
22 – Temporal horn of lateral ventricle
23 – Pulvinar nuclei of thalamus
24 – Lateral ventricle
25 – Fornix column
26 – Caudate nucleus
27 – Corpus callosum (body)
28 – Pericallosal artery
29 – Cingulate gyrus
30 – Cingulate sulcus
31 – Pineal body
32 – Internal cerebral veins
33 – Quadrigeminal cistern (cistern of
      the great cerebral vein)
34 – Tentorium cerebelli
35 – Superior colliculus
36 – Inferior colliculus
37 – Cerebral aqueduct
38 – Superior cerebellar peduncle

39 – Middle cerebellar peduncle
40 – Inferior cerebellar peduncle
41 – Cerebellar hemisphere
42 – Basal vein (Rosenthal)
43 – Anterior choroidal artery
44 – Sigmoid sinus
45 – Vertebral artery
46 – Posterior inferior cerebellar artery
47 – Cerebellomedullary cistern (Cisterna magna)
48 – Mastoid process, mastoid cells
49 – Atlanto-occipital joint
50 – Lateral atlanto-axial joint
51 – Dens of axis
52 – Axis (body)
53 – Internal jugular vein
54 – Sternocleidomastoid muscle
55 – Digastric muscle (posterior belly)
56 – Transverse ligament of atlas
57 – External auditory canal

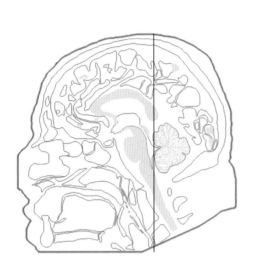

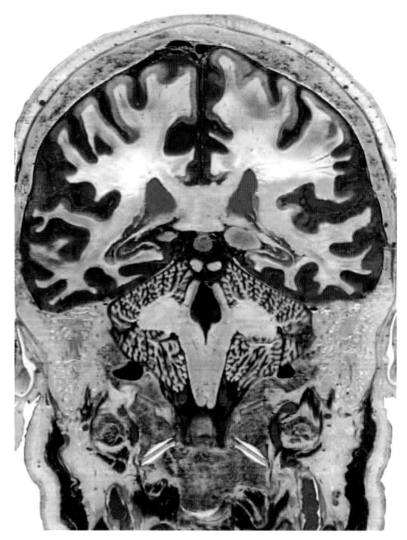

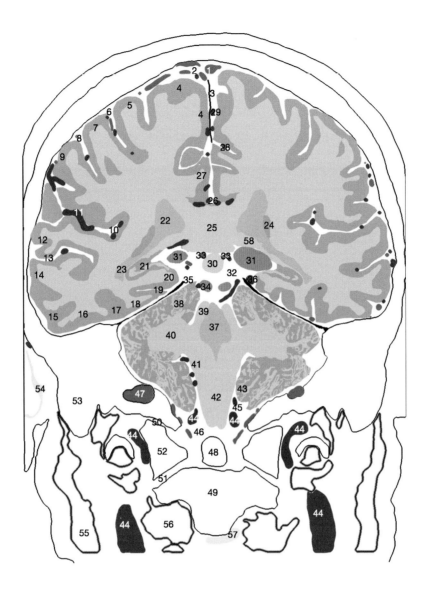

1 – Superior sagittal sinus
2 – Superior cerebral veins,
　　parietal veins
3 – Falx cerebri
4 – Paracentral lobule
5 – Precentral gyrus
6 – Central sulcus
7 – Postcentral gyrus
8 – Postcentral sulcus
9 – Supramarginal gyrus
10 – Lateral sulcus (Sylvius)
11 – Middle cerebral artery
12 – Superior temporal gyrus
13 – Superior temporal sulcus
14 – Middle temporal gyrus
15 – Inferior temporal sulcus
16 – Inferior temporal gyrus
17 – Collateral sulcus
18 – Lateral occipitotemporal gyrus
19 – Rhinal sulcus

20 – Parahippocampal gyrus
21 – Hippocampus
22 – Lateral ventricle
23 – Temporal horn of the lateral ventricle
24 – Caudate nucleus
25 – Corpus callosum (splenium)
26 – Pericallosal artery
27 – Cingulate gyrus
28 – Callosomarginal artery
29 – Paracentral artery
30 – Pineal body
31 – Pulvinar nuclei of thalamus
32 – Quadrigeminal cistern (cistern of
　　the great cerebral vein)
33 – Internal cerebral veins
34 – Inferior colliculus
35 – Tentorium cerebelli
36 – Posterior cerebral artery
37 – Fourth ventricle
38 – Cerebellar hemisphere

39 – Superior cerebellar peduncle
40 – Middle cerebellar peduncle
41 – Inferior cerebellar peduncle
42 – Medulla oblongata
43 – Cerebellar tonsil
44 – Vertebral artery
45 – Posterior inferior cerebellar artery (PICA)
46 – Cerebellomedullary cistern (cisterna magna)
47 – Sigmoid sinus
48 – Dens of axis
49 – Axis (body)
50 – Atlanto-occipital joint
51 – Lateral atlanto-axial joint
52 – Massa lateralis of atlas
53 – Mastoid process
54 – Auricular cartilage
55 – Sternocleidomastoid muscle
56 – Longus capitis muscle
57 – Intervertebral disc C2-C3
58 – Fornix (crus)

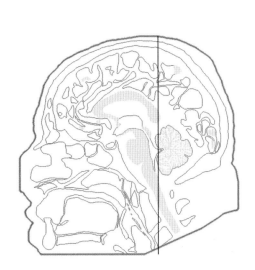

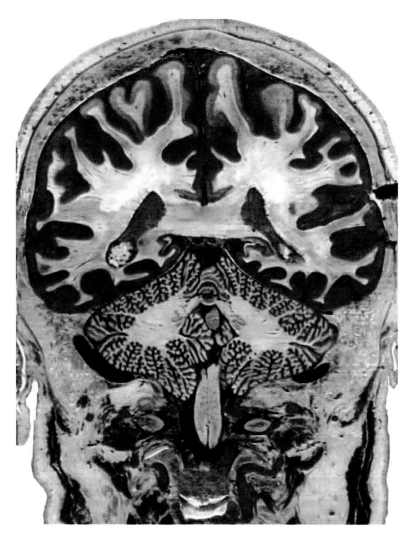

Coronal 960

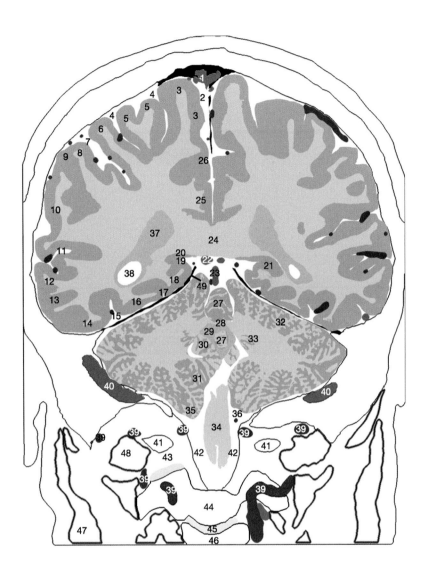

1 – Superior sagittal sinus
2 – Falx cerebri
3 – Paracentral lobule
4 – Central sulcus
5 – Precentral gyrus
6 – Postcentral gyrus
7 – Postcentral sulcus
8 – Supramarginal gyrus
9 – Lateral sulcus (Sylvius),
    posterior branch
10 – Superior temporal gyrus
11 – Superior frontal sulcus
12 – Middle temporal gyrus
13 – Inferior temporal sulcus
14 – Inferior temporal gyrus
15 – Occipitotemporal sulcus
16 – Lateral occipitotemporal gyrus

17 – Collateral sulcus
18 – Medial occipitotemporal gyrus
19 – Calcarine sulcus
20 – Fasciolar gyrus
21 – Hippocampus
22 – Internal cerebral veins
23 – Great cerebral vein (Galen)
24 – Corpus callosum (splenium)
25 – Cingulate gyrus
26 – Cingulate sulcus
27 – Cerebellar vermis
28 – Superior medullar vellum
29 – Fourth ventricle
30 – Nodulus
31 – Flocculus
32 – Cerebellar hemisphere
33 – Dentate nucleus

34 – Medulla oblongata
35 – Cerebellar tonsil
36 – Posterior inferior cerebellar artery
37 – Lateral ventricle (posterior horn)
38 – Choroid plexus
39 – Vertebral artery
40 – Sigmoid sinus
41 – Atlas (massa lateralis)
42 – Cerebellomedullary cistern
    (Cisterna magna)
43 – Lateral atlanto-axial joint
44 – Axis (body)
45 – Intervertebral disc C2-C3
46 – Vertebral body C3
47 – Sternocleidomastoid muscle
48 – Rectus capitis posterior minor muscle
49 – Tentorium cerebelli

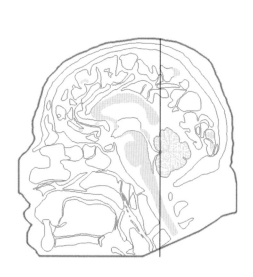

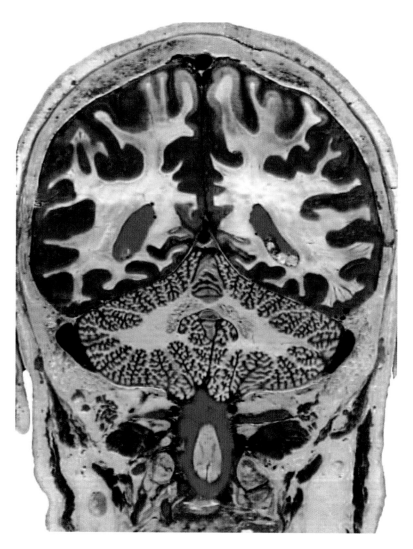

Coronal   1000

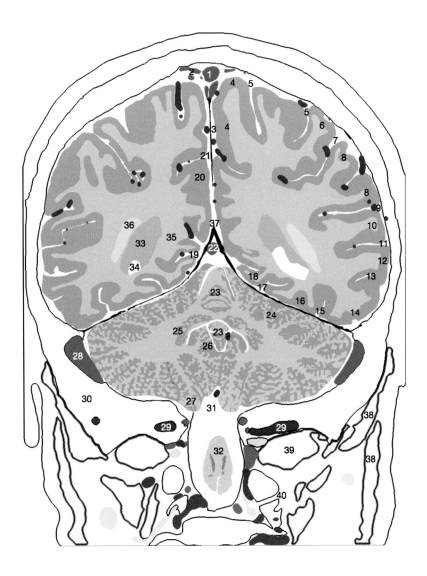

1 – Superior sagittal sinus
2 – Superior cerebral veins,
    parietal veins
3 – Falx cerebri
4 – Paracentral lobule
5 – Central sulcus
6 – Postcentral gyrus
7 – Postcentral sulcus
8 – Supramarginal gyrus
9 – Lateral sulcus (Sylvius),
    posterior branch
10 – Superior temporal gyrus
11 – Superior temporal sulcus
12 – Middle temporal gyrus
13 – Inferior temporal sulcus
14 – Inferior temporal gyrus
15 – Occipitotemporal sulcus
16 – Lateral occipitotemporal gyrus
17 – Collateral sulcus
18 – Medial occipitotemporal gyrus
19 – Calcarine sulcus
20 – Cingulate gyrus

21 – Subparietal sulcus
22 – Great cerebral vein (Galen)
23 – Cerebellar vermis
24 – Cerebellar hemisphere
25 – Dentate nucleus
26 – Nodulus
27 – Cerebellar tonsil
28 – Sigmoid sinus
29 – Vertebral artery
30 – Mastoid process
31 – Cerebellomedullary cistern
    (Cisterna magna)
32 – Medulla oblongata
33 – Lateral ventricle (posterior horn)
34 – Choroid plexus of lateral ventricle
35 – Radiation of corpus callosum
36 – Optic radiation
37 – Tentorium cerebelli
38 – Sternocleidomastoid muscle
39 – Rectus capitis posterior minor muscle
40 – Lateral atlantoaxial joint

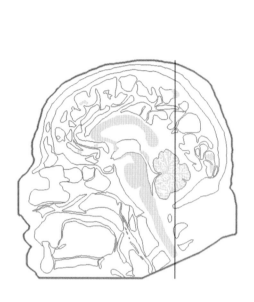

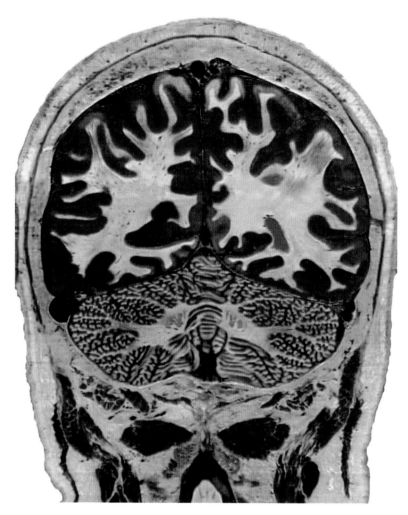

Coronal   1080

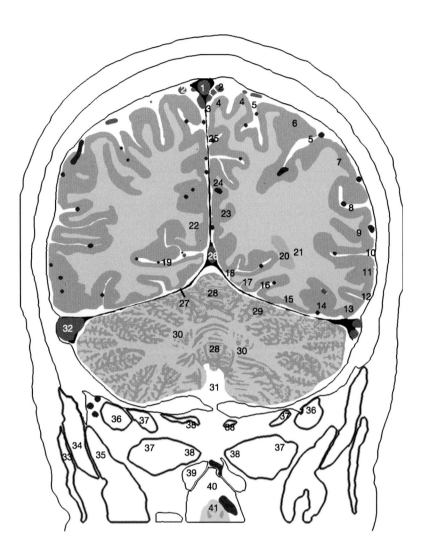

1 – Superior sagittal sinus
2 – Superior cerebral veins, parietal veins
3 – Falx cerebri
4 – Paracentral lobule
5 – Postcentral sulcus
6 – Postcentral gyrus
7 – Supramarginal gyrus
8 – Lateral sulcus (Sylvius), posterior branch
9 – Superior temporal gyrus
10 – Superior temporal sulcus
11 – Middle temporal gyrus
12 – Inferior temporal sulcus
13 – Inferior temporal gyrus
14 – Occipitotemporal sulcus
15 – Lateral occipitotemporal gyrus
16 – Collateral sulcus
17 – Medial occipitotemporal gyrus
18 – Calcarine sulcus
19 – Area striata (primary visual cortex)
20 – Lateral ventricle (posterior horn)
21 – Optic radiation

22 – Cuneus
23 – Parietooccipital sulcus
24 – Precuneus
25 – Cingulate sulcus (marginal part)
26 – Straight sinus (sinus rectus)
27 – Tentorium cerebelli
28 – Cerebellar vermis
29 – Cerebellar hemisphere
30 – Dentate nucleus
31 – Cerebellomedullary cistern (Cisterna magna)
32 – Sigmoid sinus
33 – Sternocleidomastoid muscle
34 – Longissimus capitis muscle
35 – Digastric muscle (posterior belly)
36 – Obliquus capitis superior muscle
37 – Rectus capitis posterior major muscle
38 – Rectus capitis posterior minor muscle
39 – Axis
40 – Spinal canal
41 – Spinal cord

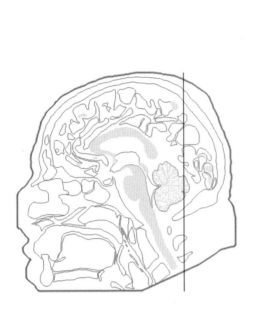

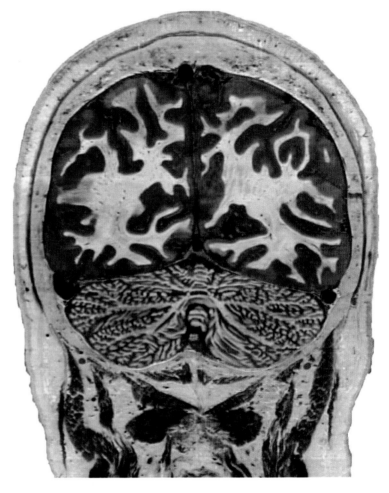

Coronal   1140

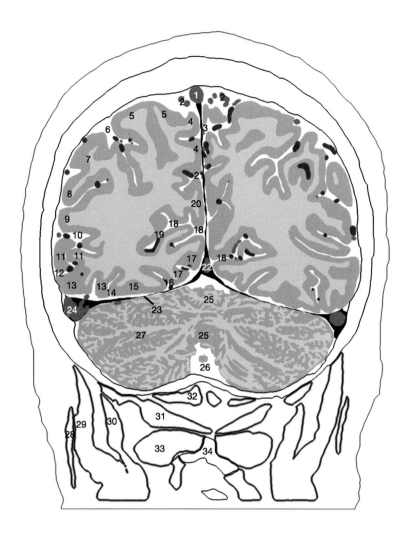

1 – Superior sagittal sinus
2 – Superior cerebral veins,
　　parietal veins
3 – Falx cerebri
4 – Precuneus
5 – Superior parietal lobule
6 – Intraparietal sulcus
7 – Inferior parietal lobule
8 – Angular gyrus
9 – Superior temporal gyrus
10 – Superior temporal sulcus
11 – Middle temporal gyrus
12 – Inferior temporal sulcus
13 – Inferior temporal gyrus
14 – Occipitotemporal sulcus
15 – Lateral occipitotemporal gyrus
16 – Collateral sulcus
17 – Medial occipitotemporal gyrus

18 – Calcarine sulcus
19 – Area striata (primary visual cortex)
20 – Cuneus
21 – Parietooccipital sulcus
22 – Straight sinus (sinus rectus)
23 – Tentorium cerebelli
24 – Sigmoid sinus
25 – Cerebellar vermis
26 – Cerebellomedullary cistern
　　(Cisterna magna)
27 – Cerebellar hemisphere
28 – Sternocleidomastoid muscle
29 – Longissimus capitis muscle
30 – Obliquus capitis superior muscle
31 – Rectus capitis posterior major muscle
32 – Rectus capitis posterior minor
　　muscle
33 – Obliquus capitis inferior muscle

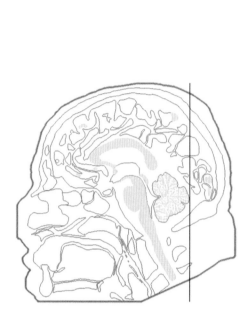

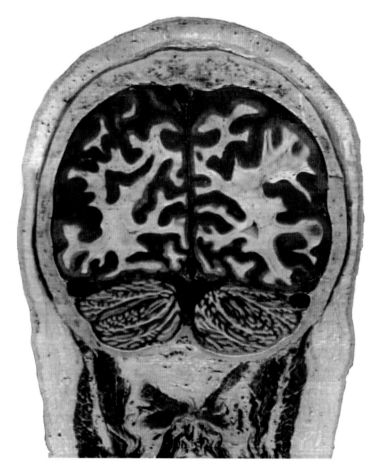

Coronal   1200

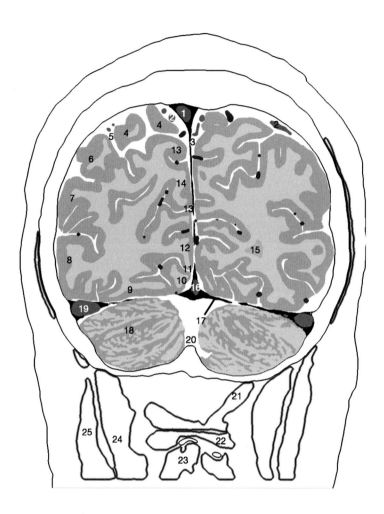

1 – Superior sagittal sinus
2 – Superior cerebra veins,
 parietal veins)
3 – Falx cerebri
4 – Superior parietal lobule
5 – Intraparietal sulcus
6 – Inferior parietal lobule
7 – Angular gyrus
8 – Occipital gyri
9 – Lateral occipitotemporal gyrus
10 – Medial occipitotemporal gyrus
11 – Calcarine sulcus
12 – Cuneus
13 – Parietooccipital sulcus

14 – Precuneus
15 – Lateral ventricle (posterior horn)
16 – Straight sinus (Sinus rectus)
17 – Tentorium cerebelli
18 – Cerebellar hemisphere
19 – Sigmoid sinus
20 – Cerebellomedullary cistern
 (Cisterna magna)
21 – Rectus capitis posterior major muscle
22 – Obliquus capitis inferior muscle
23 – Axis (spinous process)
24 – Semispinalis capitis muscle
25 – Splenius capitis muscle

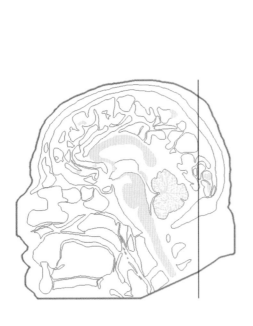

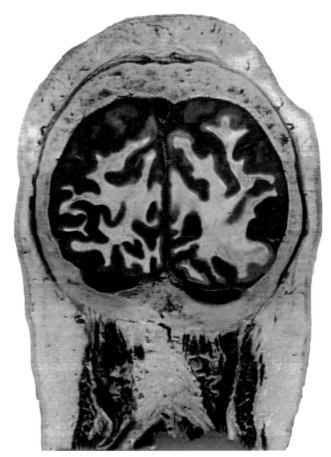

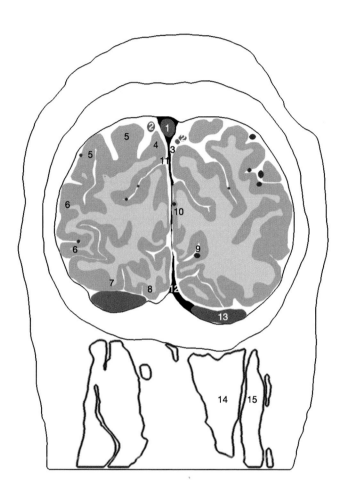

1 – Superior sagittal sinus
2 – Superior cerebral veins,
     occipital veins
3 – Falx cerebri
4 – Precuneus
5 – Angular gyrus
6 – Occipital gyri
7 – Lateral occipitotemporal gyrus

8 – Medial occipitotemporal gyrus
9 – Calcarine sulcus
10 – Cuneus
11 – Parietooccipital sulcus
12 – Tentorium cerebelli
13 – Transverse sinus
14 – Semispinalis capitis muscle
15 – Trapezius muscle

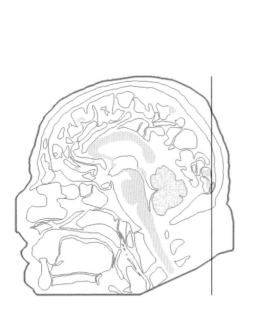
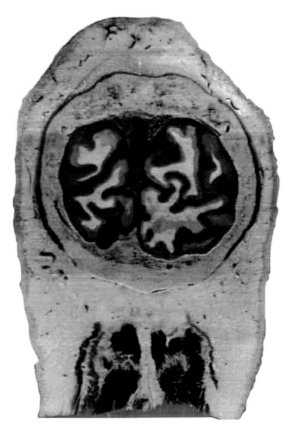

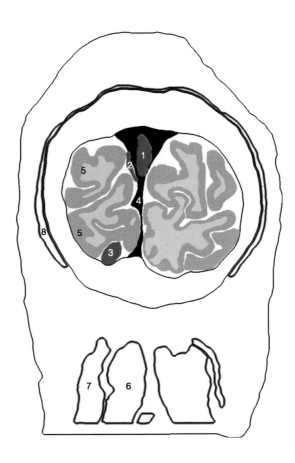

1 – Superior sagittal sinus
2 – Superior cerebral vein, occipital vein
3 – Transverse sinus
4 – Falx cerebri
5 – Occipital gyri
6 – Semispinalis capitis muscle
7 – Trapezius muscle
8 – Occipitofrontalis (epicranius) muscle (occipital belly)

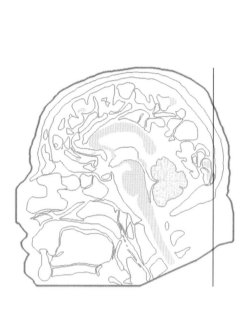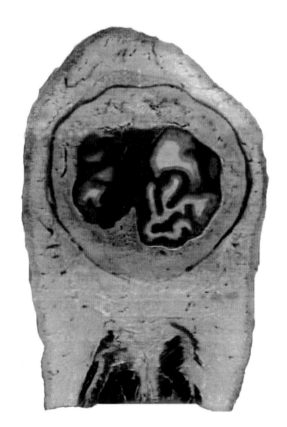

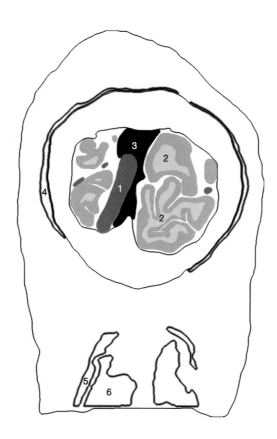

1 – Superior sagittal sinus

2 – Occipital gyri

3 – Falx cerebri

4 – Occipitofrontalis (epicranius)
    muscle (occipital belly)

5 – Trapezius muscle

6 – Semispinalis capitis muscle

3
Sagittal Sections

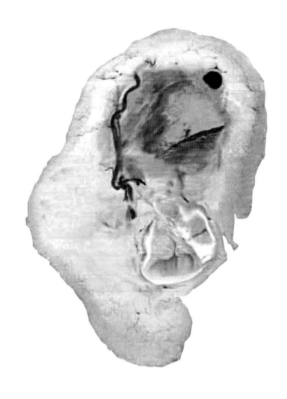

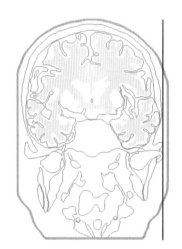

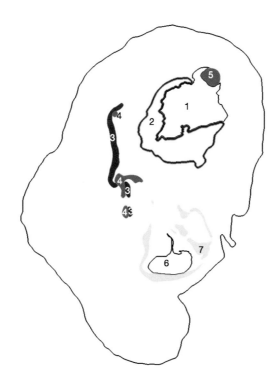

1 – Temporal bone
2 – Temporalis muscle
3 – Superficial temporal artery
4 – Superficial temporal vein
5 – Emissary vein (diploic vein)
6 – External auditory canal
7 – Auricular cartilage

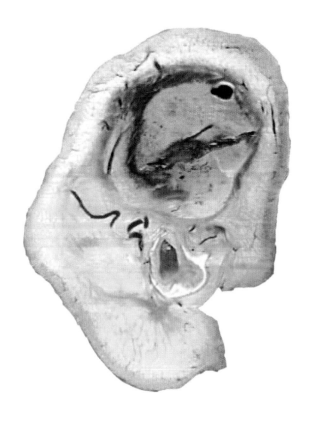

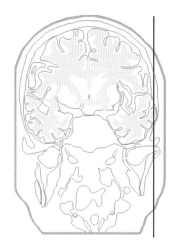

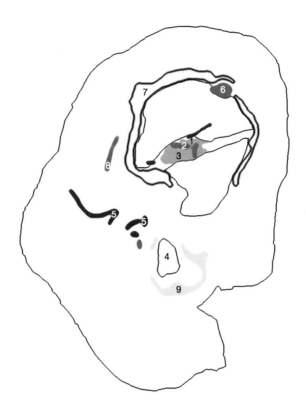

1 – Superior temporal gyrus
2 – Superior temporal sulcus
3 – Middle temporal gyrus
4 – External auditory canal
5 – Transverse facial artery
6 – Diploic vein
7 – Temporalis muscle
8 – Superficial temporal vein
9 – Auricular cartilage

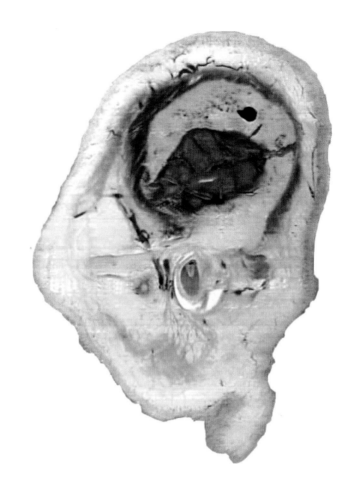

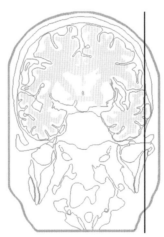

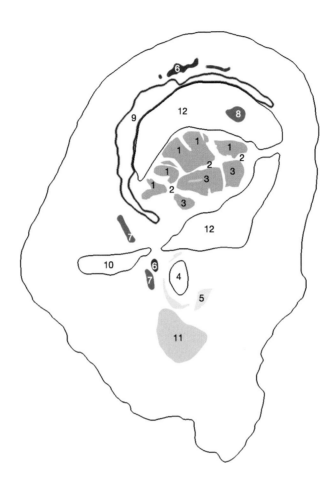

1 – Superior temporal gyrus
2 – Superior temporal sulcus
3 – Middle temporal gyrus
4 – External auditory canal
5 – Auricular cartilage
6 – Superficial temporal artery
7 – Superficial temporal vein
8 – Diploic vein
9 – Temporalis muscle
10 – Zygomatic arch
11 – Parotid gland
12 – Temporal bone

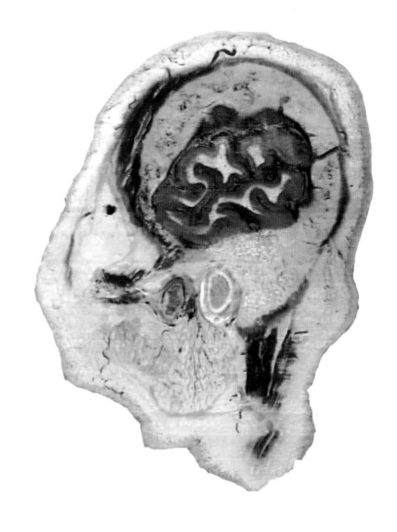

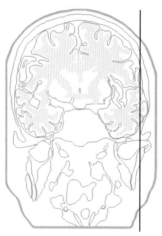

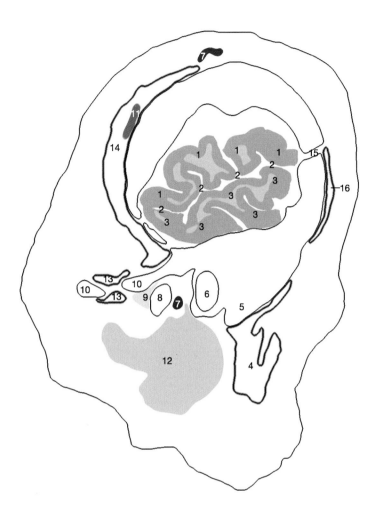

1 – Superior temporal gyrus
2 – Superior temporal sulcus
3 – Middle temporal gyrus
4 – Sternocleidomastoid muscle
5 – Mastoid process
6 – External auditory canal
7 – Superficial temporal artery
8 – Head of mandible
9 – Temporomandibular joint,
    articular disc

10 – Zygomatic arch
11 – Superficial temporal vein
12 – Parotid gland
13 – Masseter muscle
14 – Temporalis muscle
15 – Lambdoid suture
16 – Occipitofrontalis (epicranius)
     muscle (occipital belly)

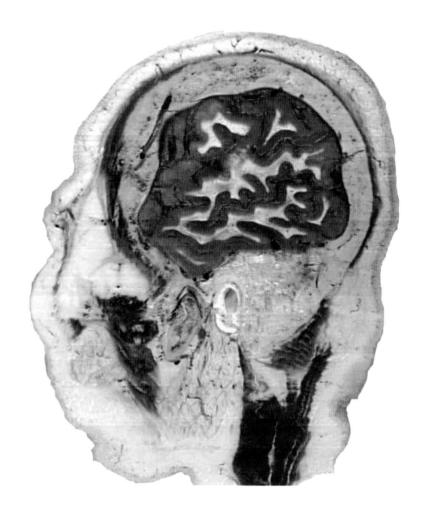

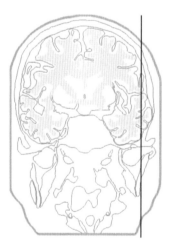

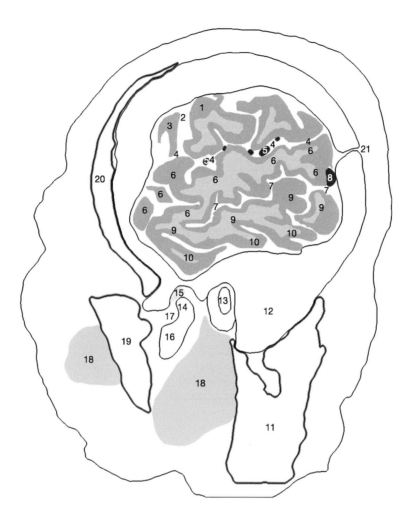

1 – Postcentral gyrus
2 – Central sulcus
3 – Precentral gyrus
4 – Lateral sulcus (Sylvius)
5 – Middle cerebral artery
6 – Superior temporal gyrus
7 – Superior temporal sulcus
8 – Middle cerebral artery
9 – Middle temporal gyrus
10 – Inferior temporal gyrus
11 – Sternocleidomastoid muscle

12 – Mastoid process, mastoid cells
13 – External acoustic meatus
14 – Head of mandible
15 – Temporomandibular joint,
    articular disc
16 – Mandible (ramus)
17 – Mandibular notch
18 – Parotid gland
19 – Masseter muscle
20 – Temporalis muscle
21 – Lambdoid suture

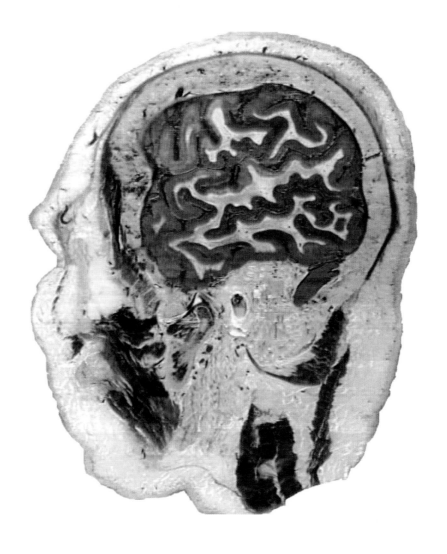

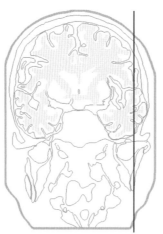

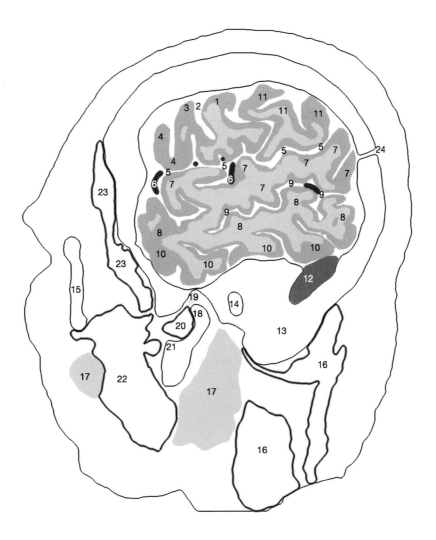

1 – Postcentral gyrus
2 – Central sulcus
3 – Precentral gyrus
4 – Inferior frontal gyrus
5 – Lateral sulcus (Sylvius)
6 – Middle cerebral artery
7 – Superior temporal gyrus
8 – Middle temporal gyrus
9 – Superior temporal sulcus
10 – Inferior temporal gyrus
11 – Supramarginal gyrus
12 – Sigmoid sinus

13 – Mastoid process, mastoid cells
14 – External acoustic meatus
15 – Zygomatic arch
16 – Sternocleidomastoid muscle
17 – Parotid gland
18 – Mandible (head)
19 – Temporomandibular joint, articular disc
20 – Lateral pterygoid muscle, lower head
21 – Base of coronoid process of mandible
22 – Masseter muscle
23 – Temporalis muscle
24 – Lambdoid suture

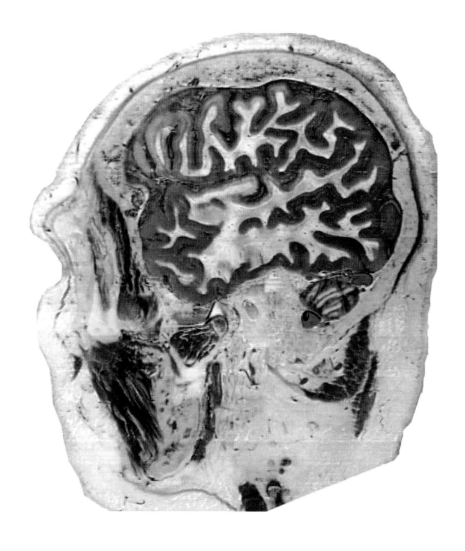

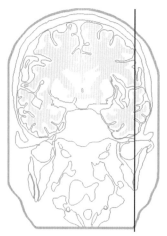

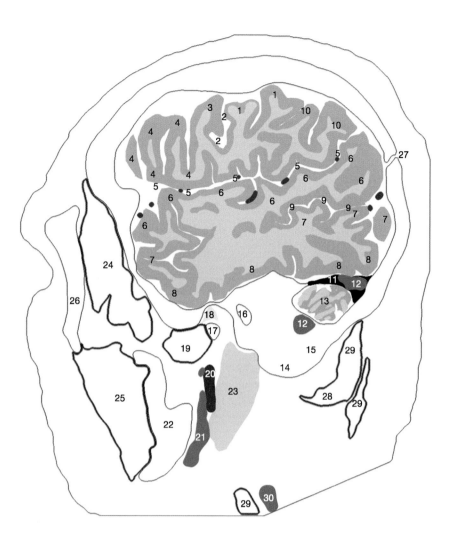

1 – Postcentral gyrus
2 – Central sulcus
3 – Precentral gyrus
4 – Inferior frontal gyrus
5 – Lateral sulcus (Sylvius)
6 – Superior temporal gyrus
7 – Middle temporal gyrus
8 – Inferior temporal gyrus
9 – Superior temporal sulcus
10 – Supramarginal gyrus
11 – Tentorium cerebelli
12 – Sigmoid sinus
13 – Cerebellar hemisphere
14 – Mastoid process
15 – Mastoid cells

16 – Middle ear
17 – Head of madible
18 – Temporomandibular joint, articular disc
19 – Lateral pterygoid muscle
20 – Common carotid artery
21 – Retromandibular vein
22 – Mandible
23 – Parotid gland
24 – Temporalis muscle
25 – Masseter muscle
26 – Zygomatic bone
27 – Lambdoid suture
28 – Longissimus capitis muscle
29 – Sternocleidomastoid muscle
30 – Internal jugular vein

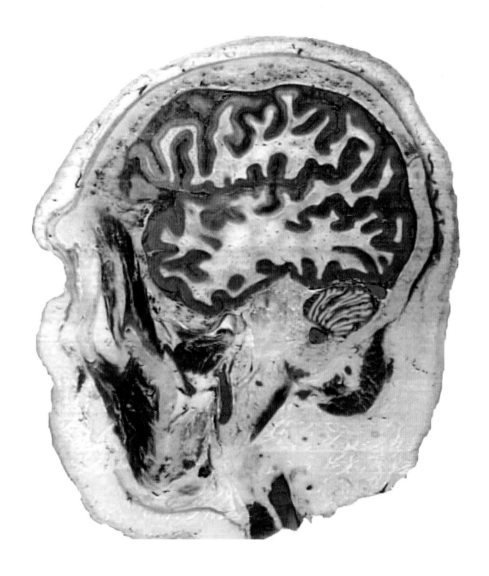

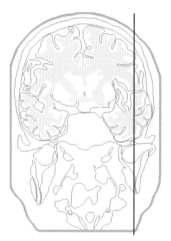

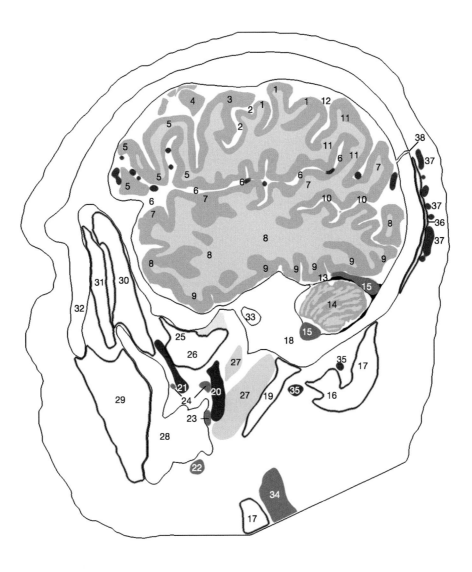

1 – Postcentral gyrus
2 – Central sulcus
3 – Precentral gyrus
4 – Middle frontal gyrus
5 – Inferior frontal gyrus
6 – Lateral sulcus (Sylvius)
7 – Superior temporal gyrus
8 – Middle temporal gyrus
9 – Inferior temporal gyrus
10 – Superior temporal sulcus
11 – Supramarginal gyrus
12 – Postcentral sulcus
13 – Tentorium cerebelli
14 – Cerebellar hemisphere
15 – Sigmoid sinus
16 – Longissimus capitis muscle
17 – Sternocleidomastoid muscle
18 – Mastoid process
19 – Digastric muscle (posterior belly)

20 – Common carotid artery
21 – Maxillary artery
22 – Facial vein
23 – Retromandibular vein
24 – Maxillary vein
25 – Lateral pterygoid muscle (upper head)
26 – Lateral pterygoid muscle (lower head)
27 – Parotid gland
28 – Mandible
29 – Masseter muscle
30 – Temporalis muscle
31 – Sphenomandibularis muscle
32 – Zygomatic bone
33 – Middle ear
34 – Internal jugular vein
35 – Stylomastoid artery
36 – Occipitofrontalis (epicranius) muscle (occipital belly)
37 – Occipital artery
38 – Lambdoid suture

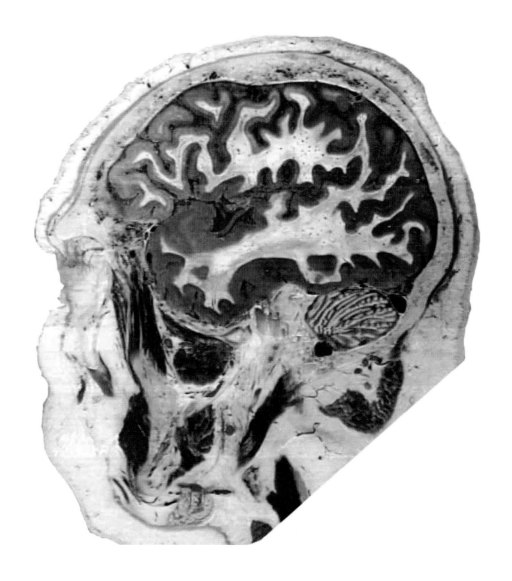

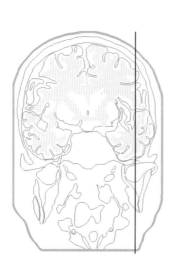

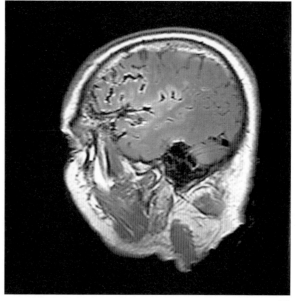

T1

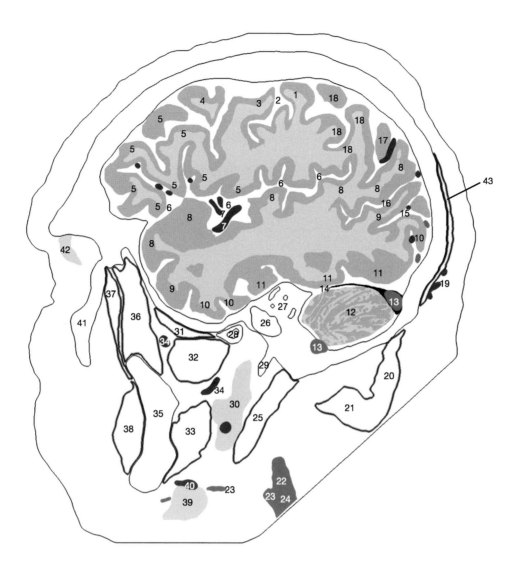

1 – Postcentral gyrus
2 – Central sulcus
3 – Precentral gyrus
4 – Middle frontal gyrus
5 – Inferior frontal gyrus
6 – Lateral sulcus (Sylvius)
7 – Middle cerebral artery
8 – Superior temporal gyrus
9 – Middle temporal gyrus
10 – Inferior temporal gyrus
11 – Lateral occipitotemporal gyrus
12 – Cerebellar hemisphere
13 – Sigmoid sinus
14 – Tentorium cerebelli
15 – Inferior temporal sulcus
16 – Superior temporal sulcus
17 – Angular gyrus
18 – Supramarginal gyrus
19 – Occipital artery
20 – Sternocleidomastoid muscle
21 – Longissimus capitis muscle
22 – Retromandibular vein
23 – Facial vein

24 – External jugular vein
25 – Digastric muscle (posterior belly)
26 – Middle ear
27 – Internal ear
28 – Pharyngotympanic (auditory) tube (Eustachio)
29 – Styloid process
30 – Parotid gland
31 – Lateral pterygoid muscle, upper head
32 – Lateral ptrygoid muscle, lower head
33 – Medial pterygoid muscle
34 – Maxillary artery
35 – Mandible
36 – Temporalis muscle
37 – Sphenomandibularis muscle
38 – Masseter muscle
39 – Submandibular gland
40 – Facial artery
41 – Zygomatic bone
42 – Lacrimal gland
43 – Occipitofrontalis (epicranius) muscle (occipital belly)

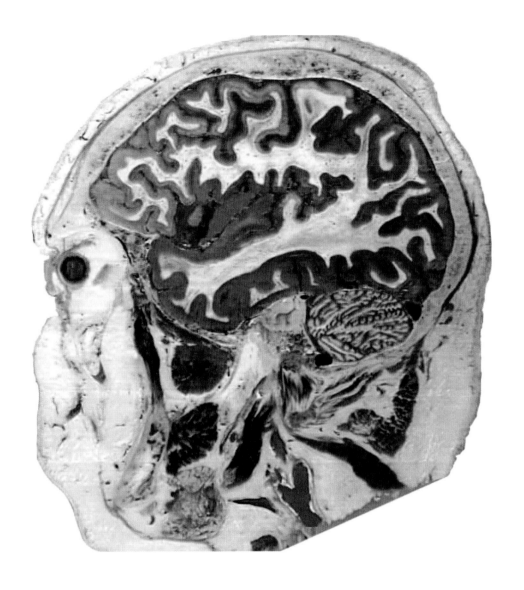

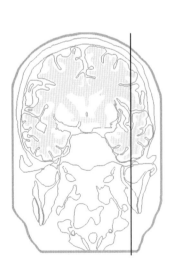

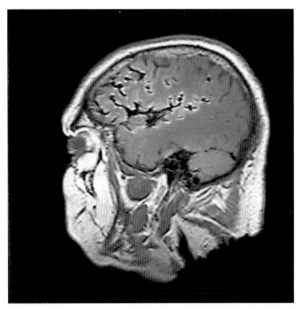

T1

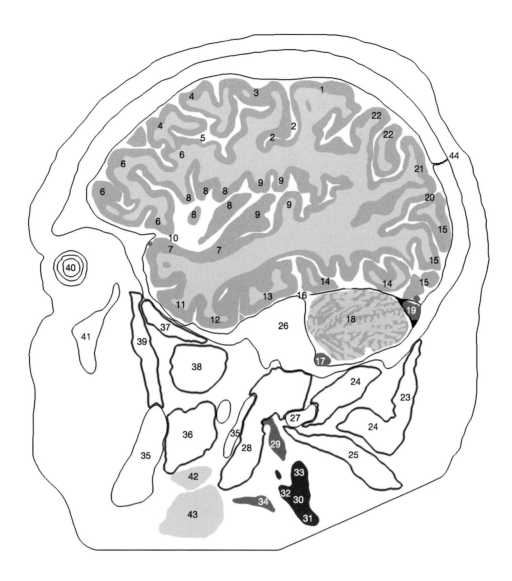

1 – Postcentral gyrus
2 – Central sulcus
3 – Precentral gyrus
4 – Middle frontal gyrus
5 – Middle frontal sulcus
6 – Inferior frontal gyrus
7 – Superior temporal gyrus
8 – Short insular gyri
9 – Long insular gyrus
10 – Lateral sulcus (Sylvius)
11 – Middle temporal gyrus
12 – Inferior temporal gyrus
13 – Lateral occipitotemporal gyrus
14 – Medial occipitotemporal gyrus
15 – Occipital gyri
16 – Tentorium cerebelli
17 – Sigmoid sinus
18 – Cerebellar hemisphere
19 – Transverse sinus
20 – Parietooccipital sulcus
21 – Angular gyrus
22 – Supramarginal gyrus

23 – Sternocleidomastoid muscle
24 – Longissimus capitis muscle
25 – Multifidus muscle
26 – Petrous bone
27 – Massa lateralis of atlas
28 – Digastric muscle (posterior belly)
29 – Retromandibular vein
30 – Carotid artery bifurcation
31 – Common carotid artery
32 – External carotid artery
33 – Internal carotid artery
34 – Facial vein
35 – Mandible
36 – Medial pterygoid muscle
37 – Lateral pterygoid muscle (upper head)
38 – Lateral pterygoid muscle (lower head)
39 – Temporalis muscle
40 – Eyeball
41 – Maxilla (zygomatic process)
42 – Sublingual gland
43 – Submandibular gland
44 – Lambdoid suture

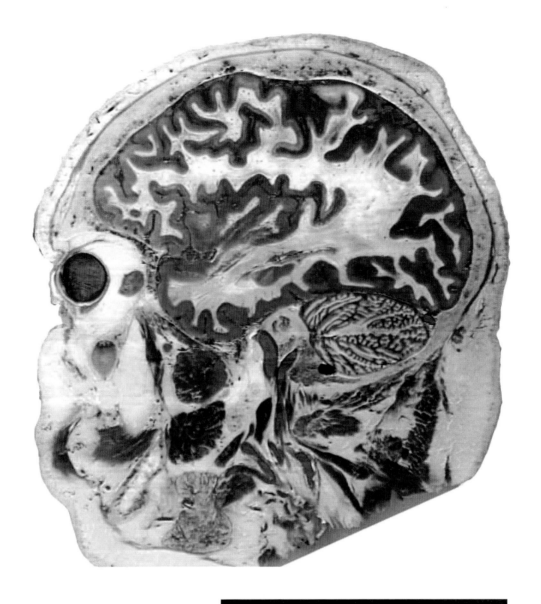

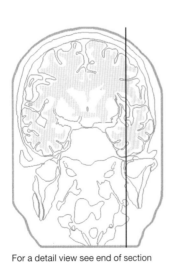

For a detail view see end of section

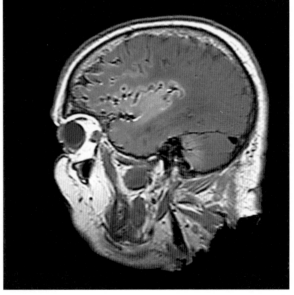

T1

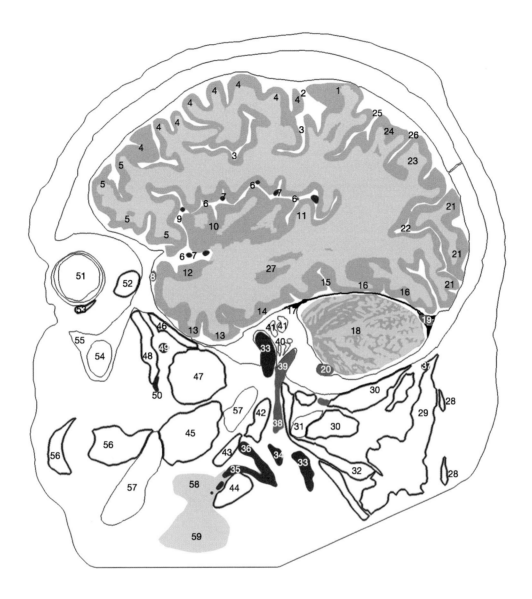

1 – Postcentral gyrus
2 – Central sulcus
3 – Superior frontal sulcus
4 – Middle frontal gyrus
5 – Inferior frontal gyrus
6 – Lateral sulcus (Sylvius)
7 – Middle cerebral artery
8 – Superficial middle cerebral vein
9 – Circular sulcus of the insula
10 – Short insular gyri
11 – Long insular gyrus
12 – Superior temporal gyrus
13 – Inferior temporal gyrus
14 – Lateral occipitotemporal gyrus
15 – Collateral sulcus
16 – Medial occipitotemporal gyrus
17 – Tentorium cerebelli
18 – Cerebellar hemisphere
19 – Transverse sinus
20 – Sigmoid sinus

21 – Occipital gyri
22 – Parietooccipital sulcus
23 – Inferior parietal lobule
24 – Superior parietal lobule
25 – Postcentral sulcus
26 – Intraparietal sulcus
27 – Hippocampus
28 – Trapezius muscle
29 – Splenius capitis muscle
30 – Obliquus capitis superior muscle
31 – Massa lateralis of atlas
32 – Multifidus muscle
33 – Internal carotid artery
34 – External carotid artery
35 – Lingual artery
36 – Facial artery
37 – Occipital artery
38 – Internal jugular vein
39 – Bulb of the jugular vein
40 – Internal acoustic meatus

41 – Internal ear
42 – Styloglossus muscle
43 – Stylohyoid muscle
44 – Digastric muscle (anterior belly)
45 – Medial pterygoid muscle
46 – Lateral pterygoid muscle (upper head)
47 – Lateral pterygoid muscle (lower head)
48 – Temporalis muscle
49 – Maxillary artery
50 – Descending palatine artery
51 – Eyeball
52 – Rectus lateralis muscle
53 – Inferior rectus muscle
54 – Maxillary sinus
55 – Maxilla
56 – Buccinator muscle
57 – Mandible
58 – Sublingual gland
59 – Submandibular gland

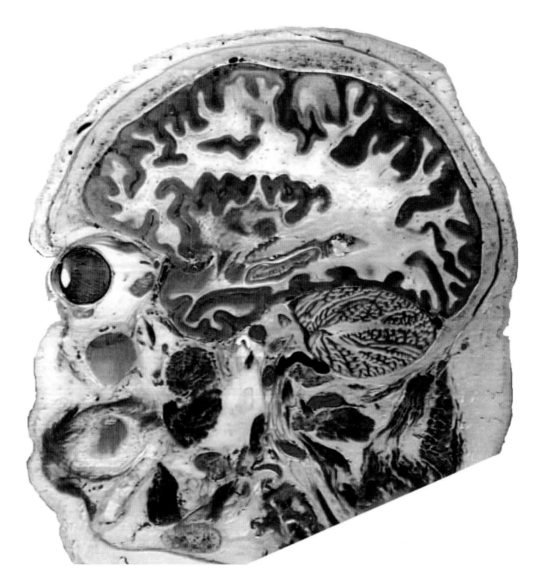

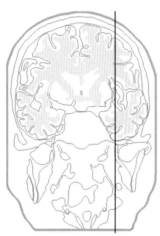

For a detail view see end of section

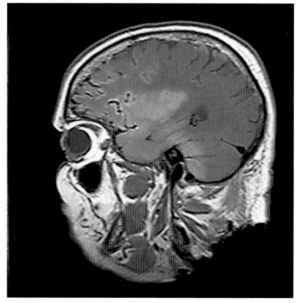

T1

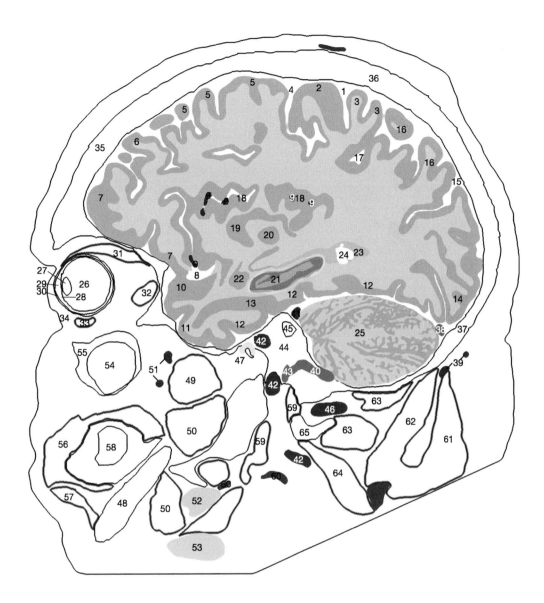

1 – Central sulcus
2 – Precentral gyrus
3 – Postcentral gyrus
4 – Precentral sulcus
5 – Superior frontal gyrus
6 – Middle frontal gyrus
7 – Inferior frontal gyrus
8 – Lateral sulcus (Sylvius)
9 – Middle cerebral artery
10 – Superior temporal gyrus
11 – Middle temporal gyrus
12 – Lateral occipitotemporal gyrus
13 – Parahippocampal gyrus
14 – Occipital gyri
15 – Parieto-occipital sulcus
16 – Superior parietal lobule
17 – Postcentral sulcus
18 – Insula
19 – Claustrum
20 – Putamen
21 – Hippocampus
22 – Amygdaloid body

23 – Lateral ventricle (occipital horn)
24 – Choroid plexus of the lateral ventricle
25 – Cerebellar hemisphere
26 – Vitreous chamber of the eye
27 – Lens
28 – Ciliary body
29 – Anterior chamber of the eye
30 – Cornea
31 – Superior rectus muscle
32 – Lateral rectus muscle
33 – Inferior rectus muscle
34 – Inferior tarsus
35 – Frontal bone
36 – Parietal bone
37 – Occipital bone
38 – Transverse sinus
39 – Occipital artery
40 – Sigmoid sinus
41 – Posterior cerebral artery
42 – Internal carotid artery
43 – Bulb of the jugular vein
44 – Petrous bone

45 – Internal ear
46 – Vertebral artery
47 – Pharyngotympanic (auditory) tube (Eustachio)
48 – Mandible
49 – Lateral pterygoid muscle
50 – Medial pterygoid muscle
51 – Maxillary artery
52 – Sublingual gland
53 – Submandibular gland
54 – Maxillary sinus
55 – Maxilla
56 – Orbicularis oris muscle
57 – Depressor labii inferioris muscle
58 – Oral cavity
59 – Stylohyoid muscle
60 – Facial artery
61 – Trapezius muscle
62 – Splenius capitis muscle
63 – Obliquus capitis superior muscle
64 – Multifidus muscle
65 – Massa lateralis of atlas

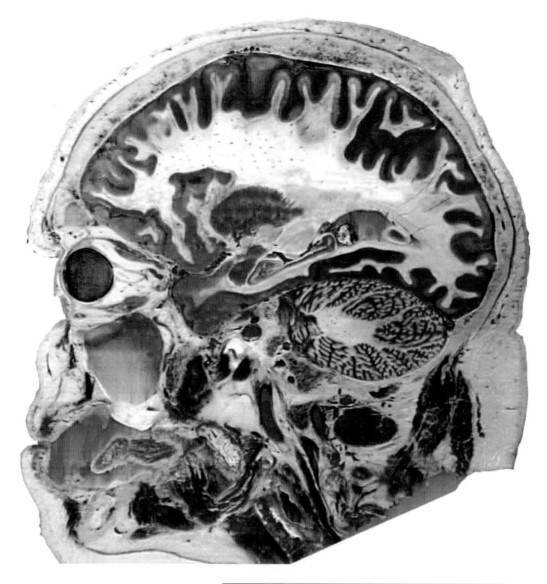

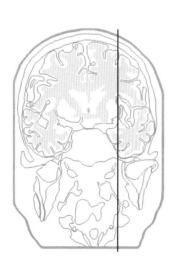

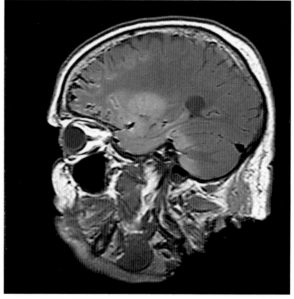

T1

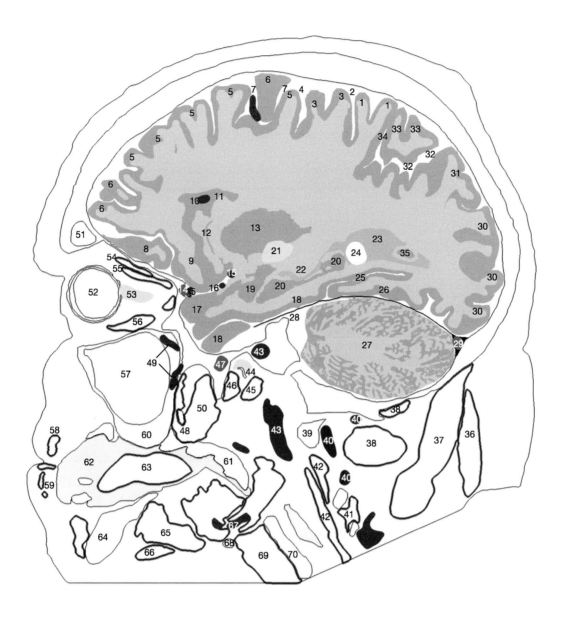

1 – Postcentral gyrus
2 – Central sulcus
3 – Precentral gyrus
4 – Precentral sulcus
5 – Middle frontal gyrus
6 – Superior frontal gyrus
7 – Superior frontal sulcus
8 – Orbital gyri
9 – Inferior frontal gyrus
10 – Circular sulcus of the insula
11 – Short insular gyri
12 – Claustrum
13 – Putamen
14 – Superficial middle
    cerebral vein
15 – Middle cerebral artery
16 – Lateral sulcus (Sylvius)
17 – Parahippocampal gyrus
18 – Lateral occipitotemporal gyrus

19 – Amygdaloid body
20 – Hippocampus
21 – Globus pallidus
22 – Lateral geniculate body
23 – Lateral ventricle (posterior
    horn)
24 – Choroid plexus of the lateral
    ventricle
25 – Collateral sulcus
26 – Medial occipitotemporal gyrus
27 – Cerebellar hemisphere
28 – Tentorium cerebelli
29 – Transverse sinus
30 – Occipital gyri
31 – Inferior parietal lobule
32 – Intraparietal sulcus
33 – Superior parietal lobule
34 – Postcentral sulcus
35 – Calcarine sulcus
36 – Trapezius muscle

37 – Splenius capitis muscle
38 – Obliquus capitis superior
    muscle
39 – Massa lateralis of the atlas
40 – Verteral artery
41 – Intervertebral joint C2-C3
42 – Prevertebral muscles (longus
    capitis, longus colli)
43 – Internal carotid artery
44 – Pharyngotympanic (auditory)
    tube (Eustachio)
44 – Levator veli palatini muscle
46 – Tensor veli palatini muscle
47 – Pterygoid venous plexus
48 – Pterygoid process
49 – Descending palatine artery
50 – Medial pterygoid muscle
51 – Frontal sinus
52 – Eyeball
53 – Optic nerve (CN II)

54 – Levator palpabrae superioris
    muscle
55 – Superior rectus muscle
56 – Inferior rectus muscle
57 – Maxillary sinus
58 – Upper lip
59 – Lower lip
60 – Maxilla (hard palate)
61 – Soft palate
62 – Oral cavity
63 – Tongue
64 – Mandible
65 – Mylohyoid muscle
66 – Digastric muscle
    (anterior belly)
67 – Lingual artery
68 – Hyoid bone
69 – Thyrohyoid muscle
70 – Thyroid cartilage

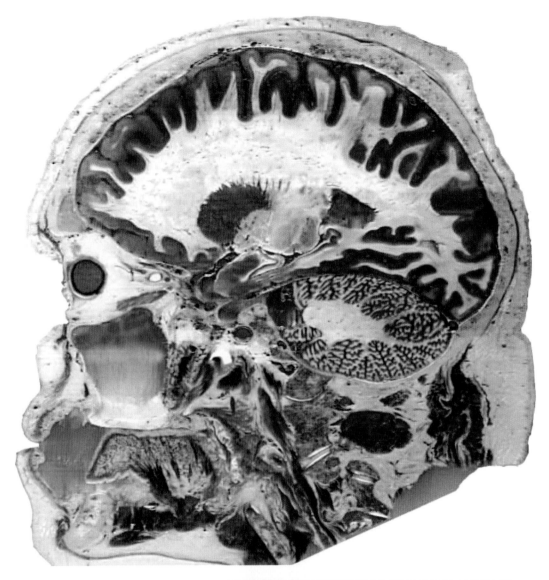

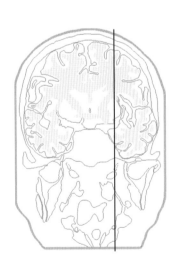

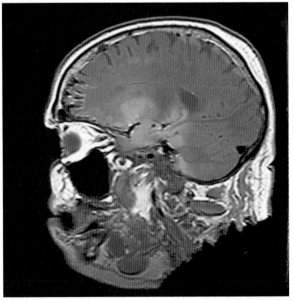

T1

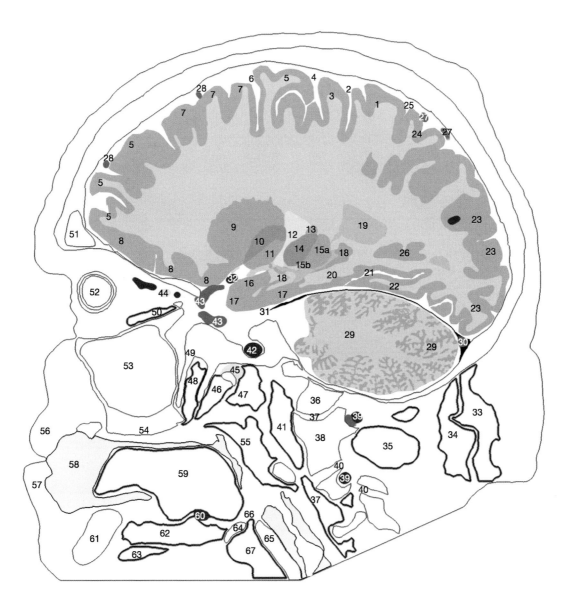

1 – Postcentral gyrus
2 – Central sulcus
3 – Precentral gyrus
4 – Precentral sulcus
5 – Superior frontal gyrus
6 – Superior frontal sulcus
7 – Middle frontal gyrus
8 – Orbital gyri
9 – Putamen
10 – Globus pallidus pars externa (GPe)
11 – Globus pallidus pars interna (GPi)
12 – Internal capsule (posterior limb)
13 – Lateral posterior nucleus of thalamus
14 – Ventral posterolateral nucleus of thalamus (VPL)
15a – Pulvinar nuclei of thalamus
15b – Medial geniculate body
16 – Amygdaloid body
17 – Parahippocampal gyrus
18 – Hippocampus
19 – Lateral ventricle (posterior horn)
20 – Lateral occipitotemporal gyrus
21 – Collateral sulcus
22 – Medial occipitotemporal gyrus

23 – Occipital gyri
24 – Superior parietal lobule
25 – Postcentral sulcus
26 – Calcarine sulcus
27 – Superior cerebral veins, parietal veins
28 – Superior cerebral veins, frontal veins
29 – Cerebellar hemisphere
30 – Transverse sinus
31 – Tentorium cerebelli
32 – Middle cerebral artery
33 – Trapezius muscle
34 – Semispinalis capitis muscle
35 – Obliquus capitis superior muscle
36 – Occipital condyle
37 – Atlantooccipital joint
38 – Atlas
39 – Vertebral artery
40 – Lateral atlantoaxial joint
41 – Longus capitis muscle
42 – Internal carotid artery
43 – Superficial middle cerebral vein
44 – Optic nerve (CN II)
45 – Pharyngotympanic (auditory) tube (Eustachio)

46 – Levator veli palatini muscle
47 – Salpyngophryngeus muscle
48 – Tensor veli palatini muscle
49 – Pterygoid process
50 – Inferior rectus muscle
51 – Frontal sinus
52 – Eyeball
53 – Maxillary sinus
54 – Hard palate
55 – Soft palate
56 – Upper lip
57 – Lower lip
58 – Oral cavity
59 – Tongue
60 – Lingual artery
61 – Mandible
62 – Mylohyoid muscle
63 – Digastric muscle (anterior belly)
64 – Hyoid bone
65 – Thyroid cartilage
66 – Thyrohyoid membrane
67 – Thyrohyoid muscle

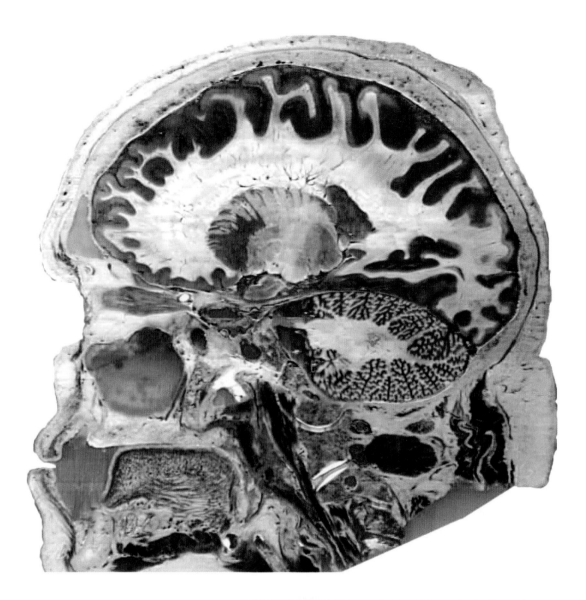

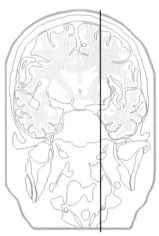

For a detail view of the basal ganglia
see end of section

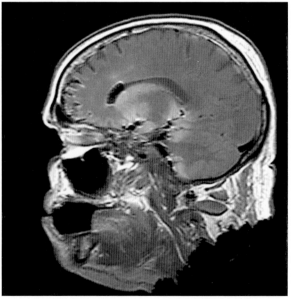

T1

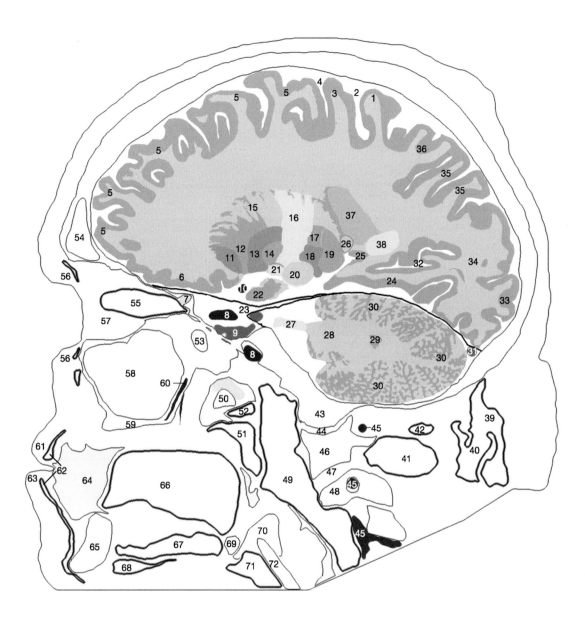

1 – Postcentral gyrus
2 – Central sulcus
3 – Precentral gyrus
4 – Precentral sulcus
5 – Superior frontal gyrus
6 – Orbital gyri
7 – Optic nerve (CN II)
8 – Internal carotid artery
9 – Cavernous sinus
10 – Middle cerebral artery
11 – Head of caudate nucleus
12 – Putamen
13 – Globus pallidus pars externa (GPe)
14 – Globus pallidus pars interna (GPi)
15 – Caudato-lenticular gray matter bridges
16 – Internal capsule
17 – Lateral posterior nucleus of thalamus

18 – Ventral posterolateral nucleus of thalamus (VPL)
19 – Pulvinar nuclei of thalamus
20 – Cerebral peduncle
21 – Optic tract
22 – Parahippocampal gyrus
23 – Tentorium cerebelli
24 – Medial occipitotemporal gyrus
25 – Hippocampus
26 – Fornix (crus)
27 – Trigeminal nerve (CN V)
28 – Middle cerebellar peduncle
29 – Dentate nucleus
30 – Cerebellar hemisphere
31 – Transverse sinus
32 – Calcarine sulcus
33 – Occipital gyri
34 – Cuneus
35 – Precuneus
36 – Superior parietal lobule

37 – Lateral ventricle (posterior horn)
38 – Corpus callosum (splenium)
39 – Trapezius muscle
40 – Semispinalis capitis muscle
41 – Obliquus capitis inferior muscle
42 – Rectus capitis posterior major muscle
43 – Occipital condyle
44 – Atlantooccipital joint
45 – Vertebral artery
46 – Atlas
47 – Lateral atlantoaxial joint
48 – Axis
49 – Prevertebral muscles (longus capitis, longus colli)
50 – Pharyngotympanic (auditory) tube (Eustachio)
51 – Soft palate
52 – Salpyngopharyngeus muscle

53 – Sphenoid sinus
54 – Frontal sinus
55 – Rectus medialis muscle
56 – Orbicularis occulis muscle
57 – Orbital fat body
58 – Maxillary sinus
59 – Hard palate
60 – Descending palatine artery
61 – Upper lip
62 – Orbicularis oris muscle
63 – Lower lip
64 – Oral cavity
65 – Mandible
66 – Tongue
67 – Geniohyoid muscle
68 – Mylohyoid muscle
69 – Hyoid bone
70 – Thyrohyoid membrane
71 – Thyrohyoid muscle
72 – Thyroid cartilage

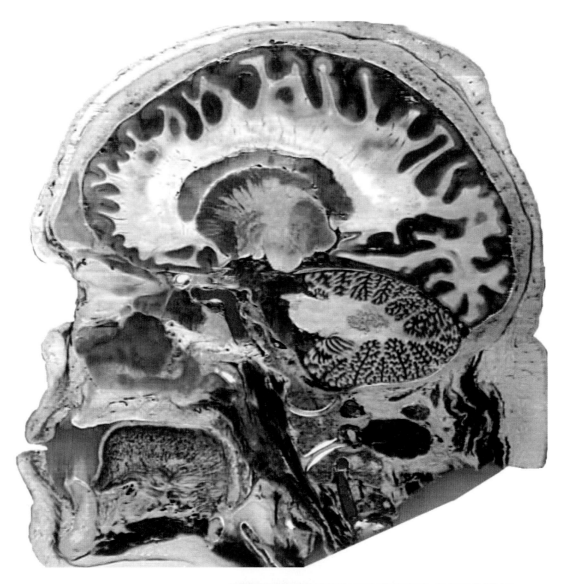

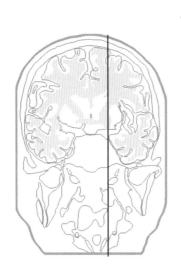

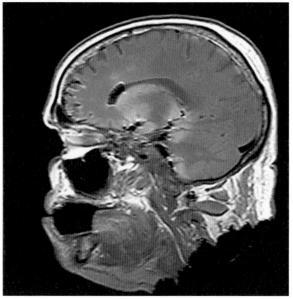

T1

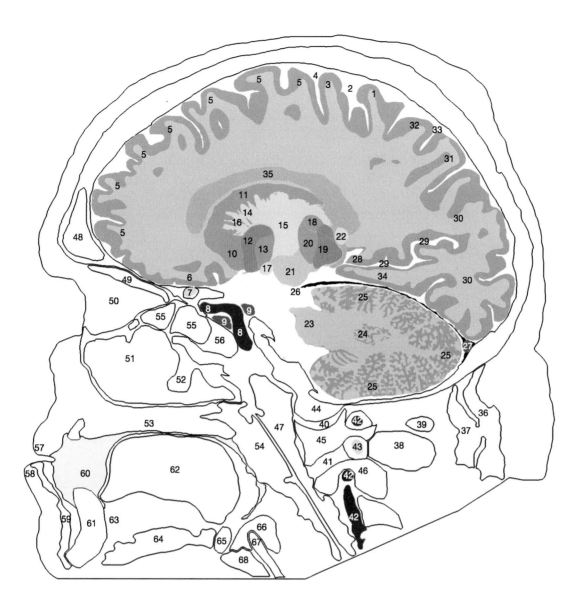

1 – Postcentral gyrus
2 – Central sulcus
3 – Precentral gyrus
4 – Precentral sulcus
5 – Superior frontal gyrus
6 – Orbital gyri
7 – Optic nerve (CN II)
8 – Internal carotid artery
9 – Cavernous sinus
10 – Head of caudate nucleus
11 – Body of caudate nucleus
12 – Globus pallidus pars externa (GPe)
13 – Globus pallidus pars interna (GPi)
14 – Internal capsule (anterior limb)
15 – Internal capsule (posterior limb)
16 – Caudato-lenticular gray matter bridges
17 – Optic tract
18 – Lateral posterolateral nucleus of thalamus
19 – Pulvinar nuclei of the thalamus
20 – Ventral posterior nucleus of thalamus
21 – Cerebral peduncle
22 – Fornix crus

23 – Middle cerebellar peduncle
24 – Dentate nucleus
25 – Cerebellar hemisphere
26 – Tentorium cerebelli
27 – Transverse sinus
28 – Hippocampus
29 – Calcarine sulcus
30 – Cuneus
31 – Precuneus
32 – Superior parietal lobule
33 – Postcentral sulcus
34 – Medial occipitotemporal gyrus
35 – Lateral ventricle
36 – Trapezius muscle
37 – Semispinalis capitis muscle
38 – Obliquus capitis inferior muscle
39 – Rectus capitis posterior major muscle
40 – Atlantoocipital joint
41 – Lateral atlantoaxial joint
42 – Vertebral artery
43 – Intervertebral foramen C1-C2, spinal nerve C2
44 – Occipital condyle
45 – Atlas

46 – Axis
47 – Prevertebral muscles (longus capitis, longus colli)
48 – Frontal sinus
49 – Superior oblique muscle
50 – Orbital fat body
51 – Maxillary sinus
52 – Inferior nasal concha
53 – Hard palate
54 – Soft palate
55 – Ethmoidal cells
56 – Sphenoid sinus
57 – Upper lip
58 – Lower lip
59 – Orbicularis oris muscle
60 – Oral cavity
61 – Mandible
62 – Tongue
63 – Sublingual gland
64 – Geniohyoid muscle
65 – Hyoid bone
66 – Thyrohyoid membrane
67 – Thyroid cartilage
68 – Thyrohyoid muscle

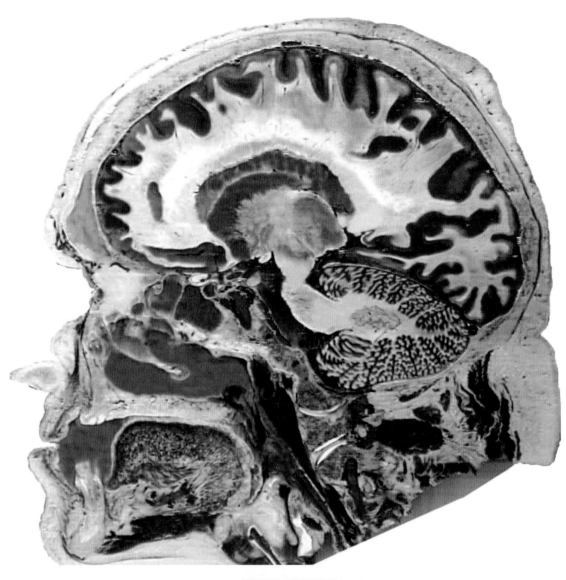

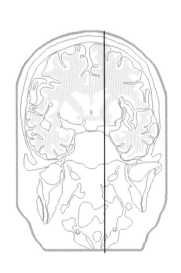

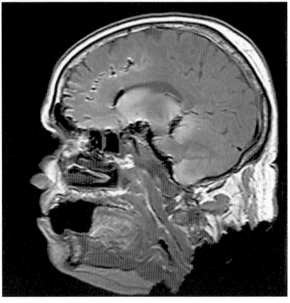

T1

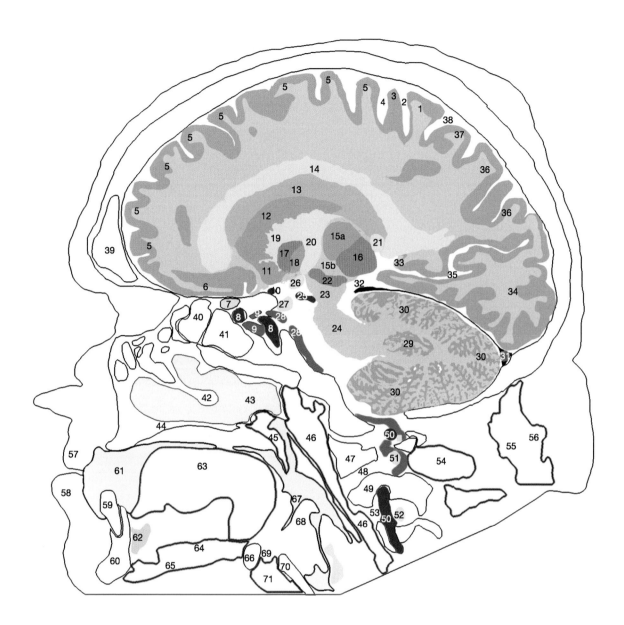

1 – Postcentral gyrus
2 – Central sulcus
3 – Precentral gyrus
4 – Precentral sulcus
5 – Superior frontal gyrus
6 – Straight gyrus (gyrus rectus)
7 – Optic nerve (CN II)
8 – Internal carotid artery
9 – Cavernous sinus
10 – Anterior cerebral artery
11 – Head of caudate nucleus
12 – Body of caudate nucleus
13 – Lateral ventricle
14 – Corpus callosum
15a – Lateral posterior nucleus
 of thalamus
15b – Ventral posteromedial
 thalamic nucleus
16 – Pulvinar nuclei of the thalamus
17 – Globus pallidus pars externa
 (GPe)

18 – Globus pallidus pars interna
 (GPi)
19 – Internal capsule (anterior
 limb)
20 – Internal capsule (posterior
 limb)
21 – Fornix (crus)
22 – Substantia nigra
23 – Midbrain (cerebral peduncle)
24 – Pons
25 – Posterior cerebral artery
26 – Optic tract
27 – Oculomotor nerve
28 – Basilar venous plexus
29 – Dentate nucleus
30 – Cerebellar hemisphere
31 – Transverse sinus
32 – Tentorium cerebelli
33 – Hippocampus
34 – Cuneus
35 – Calcarine sulcus

36 – Precuneus
37 – Superior parietal lobule
38 – Postcentral sulcus
39 – Frontal sinus
40 – Ethmoidal cells
41 – Sphenoid sinus
42 – Inferior nasal concha
43 – Nasal cavity
44 – Hard palate
45 – Soft palate
46 – Prevertebral muscles (longus
 capitis, longus colli)
47 – Massa lateralis of atlas
48 – Atlanto-occipital joint
49 – Axis
50 – Vertebral artery
51 – Intervertebral foramen C1-C2,
 spinal nerve C2
52 – Intervertebral foramen C2-C3,
 spinal nerve C3
53 –Lateral atlanto-axial joint

54 – Obliquus capitis inferior
 muscle
55 – Semispinalis
 capitis muscle
56 – Trapezius muscle
57 – Upper lip
58 – Lower lip
59 – Right inferior canine
 tooth
60 – Mandible
61 – Oral cavity
62 – Sublingual gland
63 – Body of tongue
64 – Geniohyoid muscle
65 – Mylohyoid muscle
66 – Hyoid bone
67 – Valecula
68 – Base of epiglottis
69 – Thyrohyoid membrane
70 – Thyroid cartilage
71 – Thyrohyoid muscle

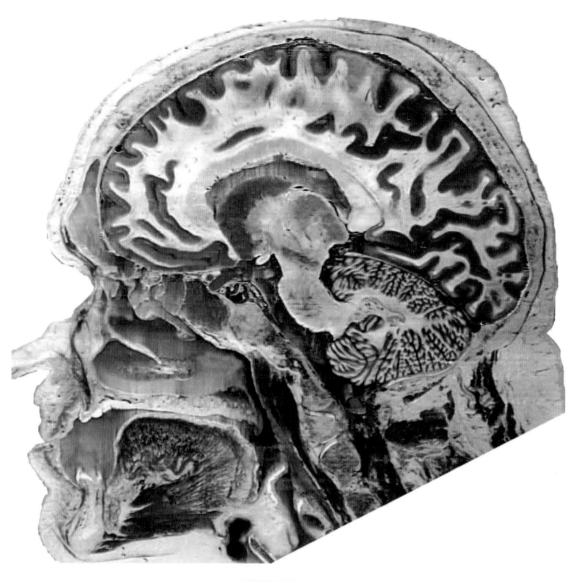

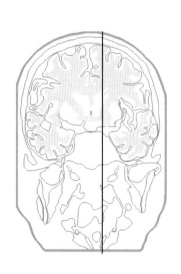

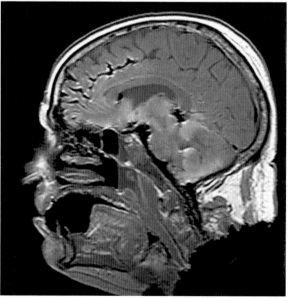

T1

Sagittal 445

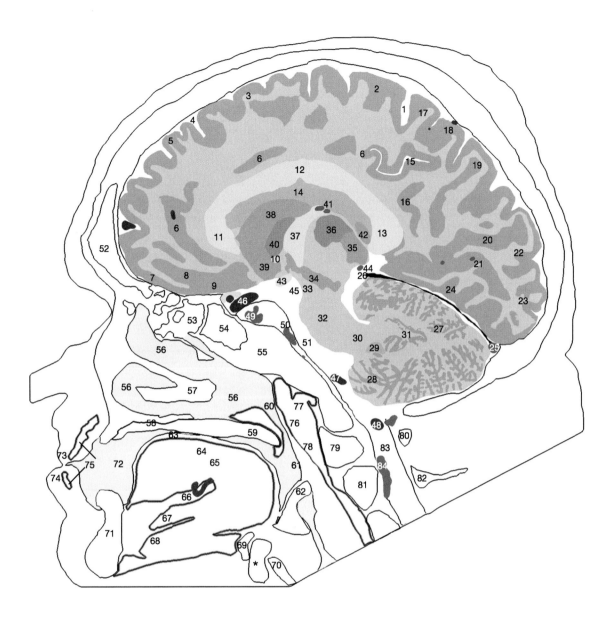

1 – Central sulcus
2 – Paracentral lobule
3 – Superior frontal gyrus
4 – Superior frontal sulcus
5 – Middle frontal gyrus
6 – Cingulate gyrus
7 – Straight gyrus (gyrus rectus)
8 – Olfactory sulcus
9 – Orbital gyri
10 – Anterior commissure
11 – Rostrum of corpus callosum
12 – Body of corpus callosum
13 – Splenium of corpus callosum
14 – Lateral ventricle
15 – Cingulate sulcus (marginal part)
16 – Subparietal sulcus
17 – Postcentral gyrus (sensory strip)
18 – Superior parietal lobule
19 – Precuneus
20 – Parieto-occipital sulcus
21 – Calcarine sulcus
22 – Cuneus

23 – Occipital gyri
24 – Medial occipito-temporal gyrus
25 – Transverse sinus
26 – Tentorium cerebelli
27 – Cerebellar hemisphere
28 – Cerebellar tonsil
29 – Fourth ventricle
30 – Middle cerebellar peduncle
31 – Dentate nucleus
32 – Pons
33 – Cerebral peduncle
34 – Substantia nigra
35 – Pulvinar of thalamus
36 – Ventral lateral nucleus of thalamus
37 – Internal capsule
38 – Body of caudate nucleus
39 – Head of caudate nucleus
40 – Globus pallidus pars externa (GPe)
41 – Thalamostriate vein
42 – Fornix (crus)
43 – Optic tract

44 – Great cerebral vein (Galen)
45 – Perimesencephalic cistern
46 – Internal carotid artery
47 – Anterior inferior cerebellar artery (AICA)
48 – Vertebral artery
49 – Cavernous sinus
50 – Basilar venous plexus
51 – Pontocerebellar cistern
52 – Frontal sinus
53 – Ethmoidal cells
54 – Sphenoid sinus
55 – Body of sphenoid bone
56 – Nasal cavity
57 – Middle nasal concha
58 – Hard palate
59 – Soft palate
60 – Rhinopharynx
61 – Oropharynx
62 – Epiglottis
63 – Tongue mucosa
64 – Superior longitudinal muscle of the tongue

65 – Vertical and transverse muscles of the tongue
66 – Lingual artery
67 – Genioglossus muscle
68 – Geniohyoid muscle
69 – Hyoid bone
70 – Thyroid cartilage
71 – Mandible (body)
72 – Oral cavity
73 – Upper lip
74 – Lower lip
75 – Orbicularis oris muscle
76 – Pharyngeal constrictor muscles
77 – Longus capitis muscle
78 – Longus colli muscle
79 – Atlas (anterior arch)
80 – Atlas (posterior arch)
81 – Body of axis
82 – Arch of axis
83 – Spinal canal
84 – Internal vertebral venous plexus
* – cyst of the thyreoglossal duct

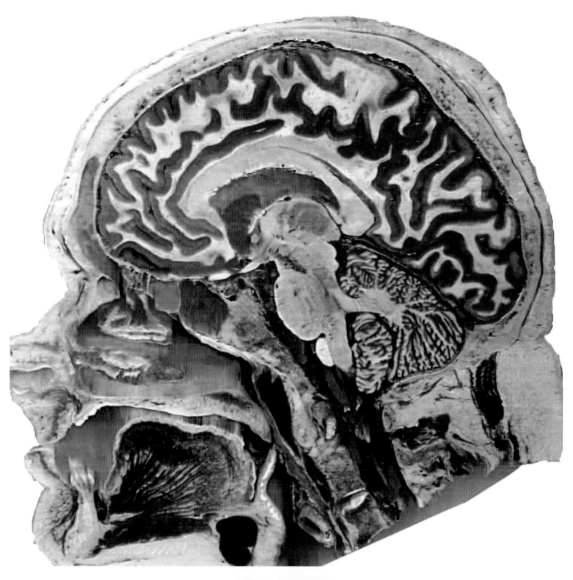

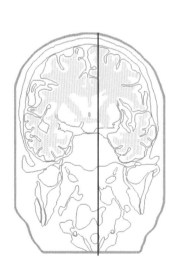

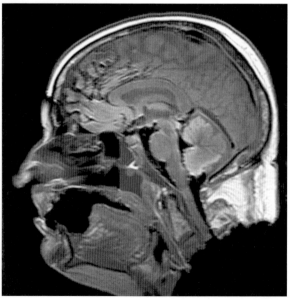

T1

Sagittal   470

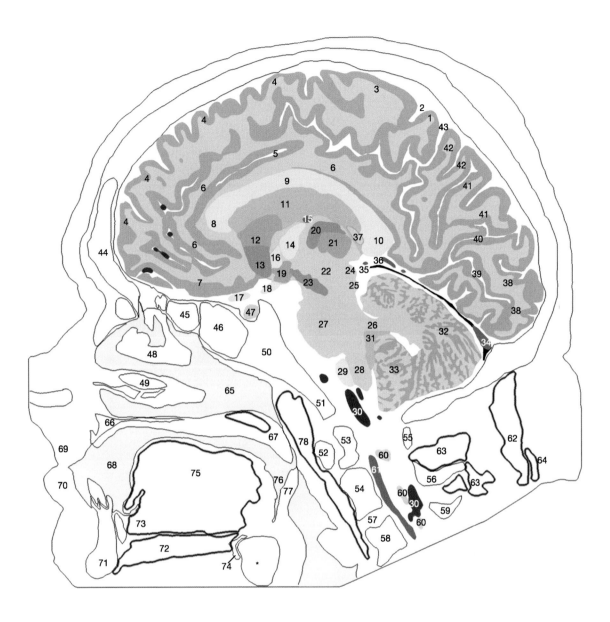

1 – Postcentral gyrus
2 – Central sulcus
3 – Precentral gyrus
4 – Superior frontal gyrus
5 – Cingulate sulcus
6 – Cingulate gyrus
7 – Straight gyrus (gyrus rectus)
8 – Rostrum of corpus callosum
9 – Body of corpus callosum
10 – Splenium of corpus callosum
11 – Lateral ventricle
12 – Head of caudate nucleus
13 – Nucleus accumbens
14 – Internal capsule (genu)
15 – Thalamostriate vein
16 – Anterior commissure
17 – Optic chiasm
18 – Optic tract
19 – Hypothalamus
20 – Anterior nucleus of thalamus
21 – Medial nucleus of thalamus

22 – Midbrain
23 – Substantia nigra
24 – Superior colliculus
25 – Inferior colliculus
26 – Superior cerebellar peduncle
27 – Pons
28 – Medulla oblongata
29 – Oliva
30 – Vertebral artery
31 – Fourth ventricle
32 – Cerebellum
33 – Cerebellar tonsil
34 – Confluence of sinuses
        (confluens sinuum)
35 – Tentorium cerebelli
36 – Great cerebral vein (Galen)
37 – Fornix (crus)
38 – Cuneus
39 – Calcarine sulcus
40 – Parietoccipital sulcus
41 – Precuneus

42 – Superior parietal lobule
43 – Postcentral sulcus
44 – Frontal sinus
45 – Ethmoidal cells
46 – Sphenoid sinus
47 – Pituitary gland
48 – Middle nasal concha
49 – Inferior nasal concha
50 – Basilar process of the
        sphenoid bone
51 – Basilar process of the
        occipital bone
52 – Anterior arch of atlas
53 – Dens of axis
54 – Body of axis
55 – Posterior arch of atlas
56 – Arch of axis
57 – Intervertebral disc C2-C3
58 – C3 vertebral body
59 – C3 vertebral arch
60 – Spinal cord

61 – Internal vertebral venous
        plexus
62 – Semispinalis capitis muscle
63 – Rectus capitis posterior
        minor muscle
64 – Trapezius muscle
65 – Nasal cavity
66 – Hard palate
67 – Soft palate
68 – Oral cavity
69 – Upper lip
70 – Lower lip
71 – Mandible
72 – Geniohyoid muscle
73 – Genioglossus muscle
74 – Hyoid bone
75 – Body of tongue
76 – Valecula
77 – Epiglottis
78 – Longus capitis muscle
* – Cyst of the thyreoglossal duct

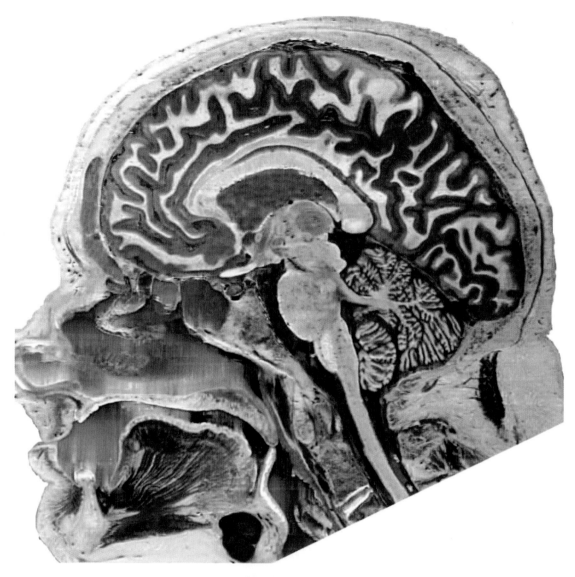

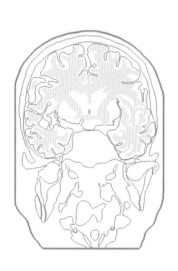

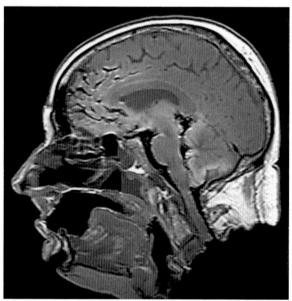

T1

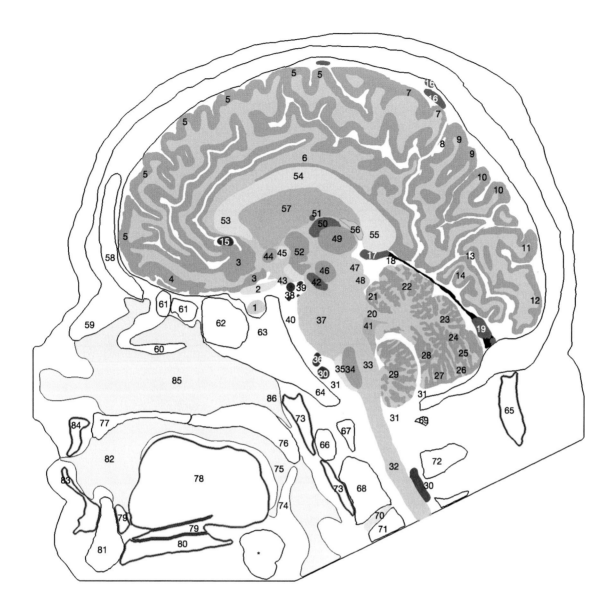

1 – Pituitary gland
2 – Optic chiasm
3 – Gyrus rectus (straight gyrus)
4 – Orbital gyri
5 – Superior frontal gyrus
6 – Cyngulate gyrus
7 – Paracentral lobule
8 – Postcentral sulcus
9 – Superior parietal lobule
10 – Precuneus
11 – Cuneus
12 – Occipital gyri
13 – Calcarine sulcus, area striata
14 – Medial occipitotemporal gyrus
15 – Pericalossal artery
16 – Superior sagittal sinus
17 – Great cerebral vein (Galen)
18 – Tentorium cerebelli
19 – Confluence of sinuses
(Confluens sinuum)
20 – Superior cerebellar peduncle
21 – Central lobule
22 – Culmen
23 – Declive

24 – Folium
25 – Tuber
26 – Pyramidal lobule
27 – Uvula
28 – Nodulus
29 – Cerebellar tonsil
30 – Vertebral artery (VA)
31 – Cerebello-medullary
cistern (Cisterna magna)
32 – Spinal cord
33 – Medulla (medulla oblongata)
34 – Oliva
35 – Pyramid
36 – Basilar artery
37 – Pons
38 – Posterior communicating
artery
39 – Interpeduncular cistern
40 – Perimesencephalic cistern
41 – Fourth ventricle
42 – Substantia nigra
43 – Mamillary body
44 – Nucleus accumbens
45 – Anterior commissure

46 – Red nucleus
47 – Superior colliculus
48 – Inferior colliculus
49 – Medial thalamic nucleus
50 – Anterior thalamic nucleus
51 – Thalamostriate vein
52 – Hypothalamus
53 – Rostrum of corpus
callosum
54 – Body of corpus callosum
55 – Splenium of corpus callosum
56 – Fornix (crus)
57 – Lateral ventricle
58 – Frontal sinus
59 – Nasal bone
60 – Middle nasal concha
61 – Ethmoidal cells
62 – Sphenoid sinus
63 – Body of sphenoid bone
64 – Basilar process of the
occipital bone
65 – Semispinalis capitis muscle
66 – Atlas (anterior arch)
67 – Dens axis

68 – Axis (body)
69 – Atlas (posterior arch)
70 – Intervertebral disc C2/C3
71 – Vertebral body C3
72 – Vertebral arch of axis
73 – Longus capitis muscle
74 – Epiglottis
75 – Valecula
76 – Soft palate (uvula)
77 – Hard palate
78 – Tongue
79 – Genioglossus muscle
80 – Geniohyoid muscle
81 – Mandilble
82 – Oral cavity
83 – Inferior lip, orbicularis oris
muscle
84 – Superior lip, orbicularis oris
muscle
85 – Nasal cavity
86 – Rhinopharynx
* – Cyst of the thyreoglossal duct

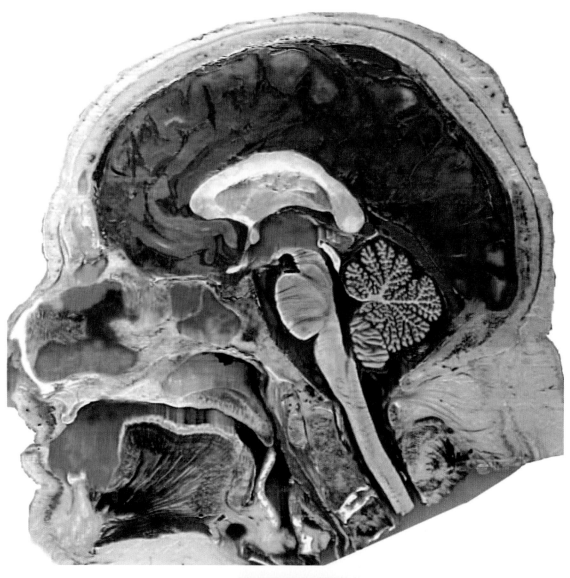

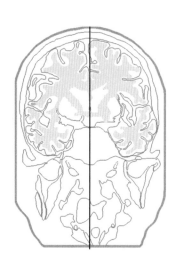

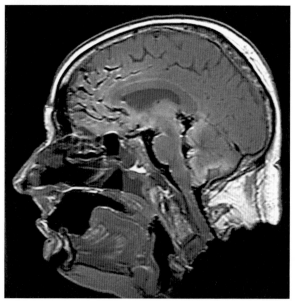

T1

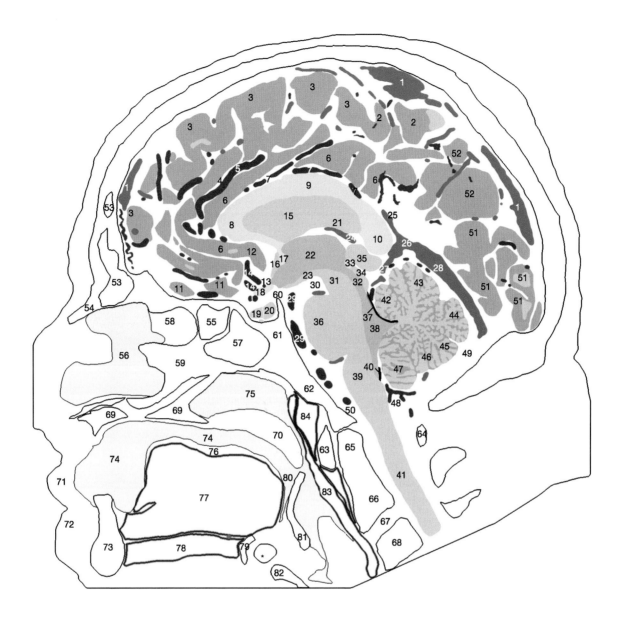

1 – Superior sagittal sinus
2 – Paracentral lobule
3 – Superior frontal gyrus
4 – Cingulate sulcus
5 – Callosomarginal artery
6 – Cingulate gyrus
7 – Pericallosal artery
8 – Corpus callosum (rostrum)
9 – Corpus callosum (body)
10 – Corpus callosum (splenium)
11 – Straight gyrus (gyrus rectus)
12 – Paraterminal gyrus
13 – Anterior communicating artery
14 – Anterior cerebral arteries
15 – Pellucid septum
16 – Lamina terminalis
17 – Anterior commissure
18 – Optic tract
19 – Anterior lobe of the pituitary gland
20 – Posterior lobe of the pituitary gland
21 – Fornix (crus)
22 – Third ventricle

23 – Mamillary body
24 – Internal cerebral vein
25 – Inferior sagittal sinus
26 – Great cerebral vein (Galen)
27 – Basal vein (Rosenthal)
28 – Straight sinus (sinus rectus)
29 – Basilar artery
30 – Interpeduncular fossa and cistern
31 – Cerebral peduncle
32 – Cerebral aqueduct
33 – Posterior commissure
34 – Quadrigeminal plate
35 – Pineal body
36 – Pons
37 – Superior medullar velum
38 – Fourth ventricle
39 – Medulla oblongata
40 – Inferior medullar velum
41 – Spinal cord
42 – Central lobule of cerebellum
43 – Culmen
44 – Declive
45 – Pyramis

46 – Uvula
47 – Cerebellar tonsil
48 – Posterior inferior cerebellar artery (PICA)
49 – Cerebellomedullary cistern (Cisterna magna)
50 – Vertebral artery
51 – Cuneus
52 – Precuneus
53 – Frontal sinus
54 – Nasal bone
55 – Ethmoidal cells
56 – Nasal cavity
57 – Sphenoid sinus
58 – Crista galli
59 – Vomer
60 – Posterior clinoid process
61 – Body of the sphenoid bone
62 – Basilar process of the occipital bone
63 – Anterior arch of the atlas
64 – Posterior arch of the atlas
65 – Dens of axis
66 – Body of axis

67 – Intervertebral disc C2-C3
68 – Vertebral body C3
69 – Hard palate
70 – Soft palate
71 – Upper lip
72 – Lower lip
73 – Mandible
74 – Oral cavity
75 – Rhinopharynx
76 – Tongue mucosa
77 – Genioglossus muscle
78 – Geniohyoid muscle
79 – Hyoid bone
80 – Valecula
81 – Epiglottis
82 – Thyroid cartilage
83 – Pharyngeal constrictor muscles
84 – Longus capitis muscle
* – Cyst of the thyreoglossal duct

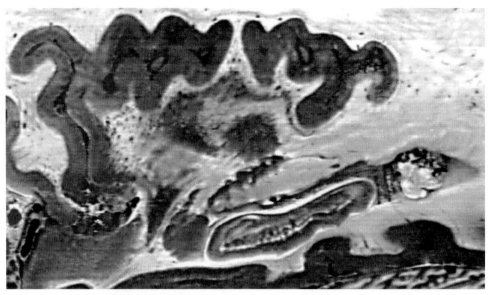

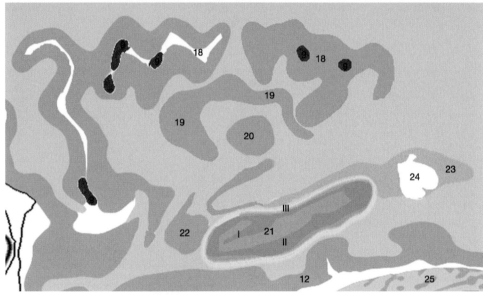

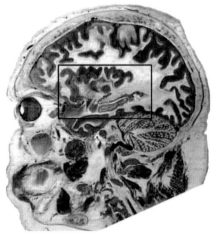

9 – Middle cerebral artery
12 – Lateral occipitotemporal gyrus
18 – Insula
19 – Claustrum
20 – Putamen
21 – Hippocampus
22 – Amygdaloid body
23 – Lateral ventricle (occipital horn)
24 – Choroid plexus of the lateral ventricle
25 – Cerebellar hemisphere
 I – Dentate gyrus
 II – Subiculum
III – Fimbria of hippocampus

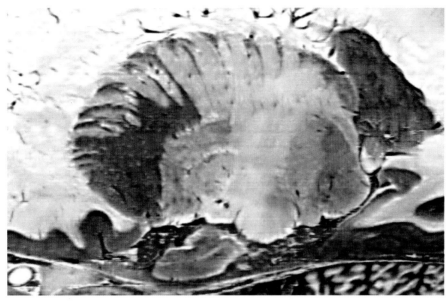

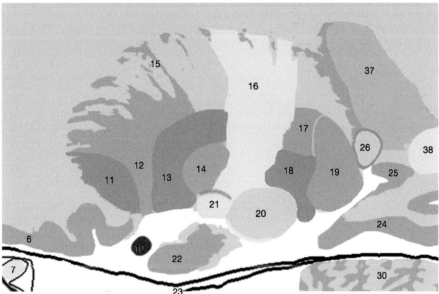

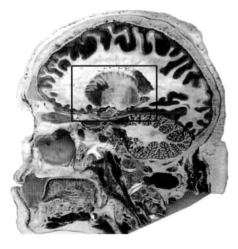

6 – Orbital gyri
7 – Optic nerve (CN II)
10 – Middle cerebral artery
11 – Head of caudate nucleus
12 – Putamen
13 – Globus pallidus pars externa (GPe)
14 - Globus pallidus pars interna (GPi)
15 - Caudato-lenticular gray matter
   bridges
16 – Internal capsule
17 – Lateral posterior nucleus of thalamus
18 – Ventral posterolateral nucleus of
   thalamus (VPL)

19 – Pulvinar nuclei of thalamus
20 – Cerebral peduncle
21 – Optic tract
22 – Parahippocampal gyrus
23 – Tentorium cerebelli
24 – Medial occipitotemporal gyrus
25 – Hippocampus
26 - Fornix (crus)
30 – Cerebellar hemisphere
37 – Lateral ventricle (posterior horn)
38 – Splenium of corpus callosum

Envoi

The consequences of relativity

The authors hope this atlas of the brain proves to be a handy tool for the students of this elusive organ. Its primary aim is pragmatic, little different from that of a road map, to help one find one's way in a city; but a map does not—nor should it attempt to—give a feel of the city's streets, its shadows, buildings, quaint, bland, exhilarating, or monumental. One might perhaps pause, at the end of the trip, to consider the queerness of the approach: looking at an incredibly complicated and convoluted organ by cutting it along three planes, utterly unrelated to any aspect of its nature.

The method is literally an application of Descartes's powerful orthogonal coordinates, the last major contribution to Euclidean geometry. Einstein conjectured that our conception of space, in which Euclidean geometry is rooted, stems from the psychological fact that we can think away the objects occupying space, but not space itself. We are inclined to ascribe space an independent existence and inherent properties that the Cartesian coordinates were designed to represent. Euclid's lasting achievement was to have rigorously derived the system of geometry, the description of these apparently inherent properties of space, from five self-evident postulates.

The fifth postulate is not quite as self-evident as the others and scholars have argued that Euclid himself might have been the first to doubt that it should be a postulate. Many a later geometer tried to derive it from the previous four, thus downgrading it to a theorem. They all failed.

Owing to the interest surrounding it, the parallel postulate has been expressed in many forms. From among the sixteen equivalent formulations listed by Heath's edition of the *Elements,* the so-called Playfair's Axiom should serve best for the present purposes: "Through a given point, only one parallel can be drawn to a given straight line."

At the beginning of the eighteenth century Giovanni Gerolamo Saccheri attempted to prove it by *reductio ad absurdum.* Assuming that either more than one parallel or none is possible, he concluded that the resulting system would yield inconsistencies. Actually, it did not, and János Bólyai and Nikolai Lobachevsky independently realized that replacing the parallel postulate by either of the two possible opposites would yield geometries that are logically consistent. Their brilliant works remained inconsequential.

Bernhard Riemann intuited that it is a question of experience to establish which geometry is true and thus what is the true nature of space. His *Habilitationschrift,* published posthumously in 1867, contains remarks worth quoting at length:

It is known that geometry assumes as things given, both the notion of space and the first principles of construction of space. She gives definitions of them which are merely nominal, while the true determinations appear in the form of axioms. The relation of these assumptions remains consequently in darkness; we neither perceive whether and how far their connection is necessary, nor *a priori,* whether it is possible. . . .

But hence flows as a necessary consequence that the propositions of geometry cannot be derived from general notions of magnitude, but the properties [of space] are only to be deduced from experience. Thus arises the problem, to discover the simplest matters of fact which suffice to determine the measure-relations of space[,] the most important system for our present purpose being that which Euclid has laid down as a foundation. These matters of fact are—like all matters of fact—not necessary, but only of empirical certainty; they are hypotheses. We may therefore investigate their probability, which within the limits of observation is of course very great, and inquire about the justice of their extension beyond the limits of observation, on the side both of the infinitely great and of the infinitely small. . . .

If we suppose that bodies exist independently of position, the curvature is everywhere constant, and it then results from astronomical measurements that it cannot be different from zero; or at any rate its reciprocal must be an area in comparison with which the range of our telescopes may be neglected. But if this independence of bodies from position does not exist, we cannot draw conclusions from metric relations of the great, to those of the infinitely small; in that case the curvature at each point may have an arbitrary value in three directions, provided that the total curvature of every measurable portion of space does not differ sensibly from zero. Still more complicated relations may exist if we no longer suppose the linear element expressible as the square root of a quadric differential. Now it seems that the empirical notions on which the metrical determinations of space are founded, the notion of a solid body and of a ray of light, cease to be valid for the infinitely small. We are therefore quite at liberty to suppose that the metric relations of space in the infinitely small do not conform to the hypotheses of geometry; and we ought in fact to suppose it, if we can thereby obtain simpler explanation of phenomena. . . .

The answer to these questions can only be got by starting from the conception of phenomena which has hitherto been justified by experience, and which Newton assumed as foundation, and by making this conception the successive changes required by facts which it cannot explain. Researches starting from general notions, like the investigation we have just made, can only be useful in preventing this work from being hampered by too narrow views, and progress in knowledge of the interdependence of things from being checked by traditional prejudices.

This leads us into the domain of another science, of physics, into which the object of this work does not allow us to go today.[1]

Non-Euclidean geometry remained a strictly mathematical pursuit for the next fifty years, until Einstein's theory of relativity showed that space is indeed non-Euclidean in nature.

Relativity theory has become accepted in its every detail as the accurate physical description of the universe, with quantum mechanics at the end of the "infinitely small" (in Riemann's words). In its technical details relativity theory remains esoteric. In 1919 Sir Arthur Eddington estimated the number of those who understand it as two; in 1988 Stephen Hawking's estimate was a few thousand, still dismally small.[2] And indeed relativity has yet to be summarized in nontechnical terms that could be absorbed in our everyday worldview, in the sense in which Copernican astronomy and Darwinian evolution inform our *Weltanschauung*, even if most people are healthily ignorant of their respective technical details.

It is generally believed that classical mechanics accurately describes how apples fall, cars roll, and planets revolve, but for objects traveling at velocities approaching that of light, terms in the equations that were hitherto negligible become significant, or vice versa; that Einstein's formulas take the form of Newton's when the velocities of bodies in motion are low enough for certain components of the relativistic formulas to vanish. In other words, classical mechanics is said to be a "special case" of relativity. On the geometrical side, we learn that space is "curved," so to speak, over the unfathomable galactic distances but only slightly so within our solar system (four seconds of an arc per century is a puny difference, after all, between the measured revolution of Mercury and the one predicted by Newtonian physics). Over terrestrial distances, one can safely rely on Euclid's triangles (and, in fact, for most of our earthly business we can even ignore the Copernican revolution, as land surveyors still do, with no

1. Bernhard Riemann, "On the hypotheses which lie at the bases of geometry," trans. William Kindgdon Clifford, *Nature*, 8 (1873), no. 183, 184: 14–17, 36, 37. Translation slightly emended.

2. It is instructive to quote Chaim Weizmann and Isaiah Berlin here. Weizmann wrote: "Einstein explained his theory to me every day, and soon I was fully convinced that he understood it." Berlin: "Albert Einstein's chief title to immortal fame is his transcendent scientific genius, about which, like the vast majority of mankind, I am totally incompetent to speak." Neither author had particularly modest cognitive abilities nor was exceedingly modest about them.

prejudice to their professional performance). As a consequence, Newtonian mechanics and Euclidean geometry are still taught through high school and college without qualifications, and our intuition of space has remained untouched by non-Euclidean geometry in the sense in which, once the Copernican revolution has been assimilated, we unflinchingly acknowledge that, contrary to what we see, it is not the sun that goes down at dusk, behind the hills.

A careful consideration of the matter, along with a few but noteworthy commentators, suggests otherwise. Bertrand Russell in 1926 was probably the first to point out that Einstein's arguments undermine Newtonian physics and "would have remained valid even if his own law of gravitation had not proved right."[3] Later (in *The Structure of Scientific Revolutions*), Thomas S. Kuhn also noted that relativity invalidated classical mechanics, but this contention was obscured by the dust his seminal little book stirred in other respects.

In spite of these and a few other exegetes, and in spite of relativity being proved correct with every development of physics and technology (including the global positioning system, which must very rigorously account for relativistic time contraction), we were content to go on believing that geometry is true, parallel lines are parallel, and the sum of the angles in a triangle is equal to two right angles, at least here and now. General relativity remained even more nebulous and we can read in popular expositions how the mysterious gravity, an instantaneous action at a distance between two bodies, has been explained away as a no less mysterious consequence of the intuitively meaningless notion of curvature of space-time. A better take-home lesson would be that relativity has shown *how* space is, so

far as physics can ascertain, and that it is certainly *not* Euclidean.

Toward a non-Euclidean anatomy

Because the principles of biology cannot analytically be derived from physics, neither should it be assumed that the nature of biological space must necessarily emulate that of physical space.

In these concluding remarks to an atlas of cross-sectional anatomy, I wish to take stock—or to propose that we take stock—of non-Euclidean geometry, insofar as it concerns our humble trade.

The story of space goes like this: our intuition gives rise in its most abstract and most general form to geometry. But geometry is being undermined on two fronts. Internally, it has been revealed that geometry remains consistent if counterintuitive assumptions are admitted. The notion that we cannot *a priori* know the nature of space but that it is a matter of experience is reinforced. Then, from outside geometry, physics tells us its minimum requirements, which we can better appreciate if we remember that physics itself is an abstraction that reduces bodies to nondeformable object points.

We are thus authorized, indeed, summoned to carry over the doubts raised regarding the nature of space into biology, along with the tools and useful pointers that may help us to understand how space *might* be.

Anatomy has a dual nature. On one hand, its most immediate aims seem to justify Hegel's scorn of "the knowledge of the parts of the body regarded as lifeless, we are quite sure that we do not yet possess the subject matter itself, the content of this science, but must concern ourselves with the particulars. This is an aggregate of information with no right to bear the name of science."[4] Even this admittedly modest aim is increas-

---

3. "[W]hen two bodies are in relative motion, like the sun and a planet, there is no such physical fact as 'the distance between the bodies at a given time'; this alone shows that Newton's law of gravitation is logically faulty. Fortunately, Einstein has not only pointed out the defect, but remedied it. His arguments against Newton, however, would have remained valid even if his own law of gravitation had not proved right." Bertrand Russell, "Philosophical Consequences of Relativity," *Encyclopaedia Britannica*, 13th ed. (1926).

4. G. W. F. Hegel, "Preface. On scientific knowing," in *The Phenomenology of Mind*, trans. J. B. Baillie (New York: Harper and Row, 1967), p. 67. The translation has been slightly emended and the fragment edited for clarity.

ingly proving beyond reach, especially as the latter developments of minimally invasive medicine demand quantitative knowledge, about which more later.

A loftier aim—nowadays less visible and more intertwined with the aims of other branches of science, biology, taxonomy, anthropology, once optimistically regarded as crucial for physiology (and this trend is bound to return)—is for anatomy to provide a key, at least a clue, for understanding function, evolution, meaning in a biological sense. Embryology used to be regarded as the key to or at least an essential part of the answer to the question of biological meaning. The best expression of this effort materialized in the oft-praised, less often read, even less appreciated (also by this author) thousand pages of D'Arcy Thompson's dense and learned *On Growth and Form* (1917). The fact that Thompson's focus has not grown into a scientific trend is symptomatic, as is the fact that in spite of unabated praise only an abridged version is now in print.

The brain can be seen as the hypertrophied proximal end of the central nervous system, a tumor at the end of a swollen tube; as such it is still part of the neural tube of embryological development, which is very much a midline, lengthwise warping of the same ectoderm that will give rise to a wide variety of unrelated structures: the skin, hair, nails, even the enamel of the teeth.

The hemispheres of the brain can be regarded as a failure of the neural crests to fuse, and the *grande complication* of the sulci and gyri may be seen as the result of stuffing a large balloon into the much smaller receptacle of the skull. To borrow the wording of a thinker of disreputable memory, this describes the process in logical, not chronological, order, as is true of explanations of other embryological processes of perplexing complexity.

All this has been known and described to the extent that it has been possible and deemed necessary or worthwhile. It had long been an advantage and a hindrance at the same time that anatomy and hence (indirectly) embryology were ancillaries to medicine, which itself is not a pure science but an application and an effort to manipulate nature, therefore more akin to engineering than to physics. And the stern basic disciplines were cultivated only insofar as a more or less profitable result could be counted upon.

What non-Euclidean geometry and its ample validation by physics can contribute is the recognition that studying the process of organogenesis and its result as embodied in the adult anatomy, especially its quantification, is bound to be more successful after the Cartesian heresy has been abandoned.

At this particular point, the gratuitous cultivation of science for the sake of knowledge intersects with the pragmatic needs of anatomy as *ancilla medicinae*. Modern interventional techniques have become possible, thanks to the development of magnetic resonance imaging and micro- and nanotechnology. Minimally invasive techniques are a promising approach to clinical procedures, for they allow access to internal organs through tiny breaches or without any openings of the body's natural barriers.

Techniques for producing a detailed image of an individual body and entering the body by means of extremely small instruments are now available. Both prevent the human observer, the clinician, from navigating with the aid of one's senses as clinicians traditionally have done. Image guidance requires a computer-readable version of anatomical knowledge, as well as quantification to an unprecedented degree of accuracy. And with this we arrived at a bottleneck, the same point at which traditional descriptive anatomy has found itself.

A cursory look at any textbook will reveal the stage at which quantitative description was arrested, and anyone familiar with medical image analysis can confirm how useless traditional shape description and measurements proved to be. It was practical to say that the kidney is bean-shaped so long as this was meant to train a physician to recognize the organ, but it became as meaningless as to say that beans are kidney-shaped as soon as one attempted to translate this knowledge into the language of computers or (earlier, but this was less evident then) to see the shape's relevance for its function. It was witty and effective to name the hippocampus after the seahorse it resembles, but the name proved impotent in the effort to create an algorithm to recognize the organ's intricate shape.

In order to illustrate the problems encountered when anatomy tackles quantification, we may look at the standard description of a relatively simple organ, the aorta.

The ascending aorta, about 5 cm long, begins at the base of the left ventricle, level with the third left costal cartilage's lower border. At its origin, close to the aortic annulus, the sectional profile is larger and not circular because of three hemispherical outward bulges (sinuses of Valsalva), one posterior (non-coronary), one left and one right, which correspond to the three cusps of the aortic valve. Distal to the aortic annulus are three aortic sinuses, beyond which the vessel's callibre is slightly increased by a bulging of its right wall; this aortic bulb gives the vessel an oval section.[5]

On this basis it has not been possible to achieve a good quantitative description of anatomy, much less to apply it in computational image analysis.

The reason is the unsuitability of the Euclidean metrics, not unlike the unsuitability of pliers for loosening a bolt. Some bolts will yield, some will be stripped by the crude mismatch, but most require a wrench.

The first lesson of non-Euclidean geometry is that while things may be convoluted, it is no less legitimate to consider them straight and space convoluted. Einstein left us with no doubt that the question whether space is Euclidean, Riemannian, or any other structure should not be decided on the basis of convenience[6].

5. *Gray's Anatomy: The Anatomical Basis of Medicine and Surgery,* 38th ed., Peter L. Williams, Chairman of the Editorial Board (London: Churchill Livingstone, 1995), p. 1505.

6. "On the basis of the general theory of relativity . . . space as opposed to 'what fills space' which is dependent of the co-ordinates has no separate existence . . . the question whether this continuum has a Euclidian, Riemannian or any other structure is a question of physics proper, which must be answered by experience, and not a question of a convention to be chosen on grounds of mere expediency." Albert Einstein, "Geometry and Experience," Lecture before the Prussian Academy of Sciences, 1921, in *Ideas and Opinions,* (New York: Three Rivers Press, Crown Publishers, Inc., 1982), p. 238.

True, in order to apply this lesson to anatomy, one must first subject one's mind to a more radical twist than the gentle bend of a ray of light grazing the sun. Moreover, one must likely give up another assumption, not questioned by physics, the homogeneity of space—although when Einstein wrote that space as opposed to what fills space has no independent existence, the question was implicitly asked.

Thus equipped, we can proceed to viewing the embryonic disc as a quasi-Euclidean solid—if only for an instant—for it already has three layers that will momentarily start their contorted dance. At first, the layers share a coordinate system and a common clock, and it is conceivable to consider invariant not their coordinate system but their existence, and to modify the coordinate system according to the change in their shape and differentiation. As the layers change we will end up with a vast number of coordinate systems and metrics corresponding to the different organ systems, which is disconcerting at first, but the following *excursus* may help to ease the difficulty.

Edwin Abbott's *Flatland* is popular probably because it stretches and nimbles the mind. Just as a reader can relate to those unfortunate two-dimensional creatures for whom our matter-of-fact third dimension is such a great leap, we can fathom, albeit not picture, a world of four dimensions, or so the fans of *Flatland* feel.

In the same vein, we should first imagine the human anatomy "unfurled" about one organ at a time, as illustrated in Figure 1: first around, say, the spine (A and B), and then about the aorta (C and D). Figure 2 is meant to illustrate this exercise in more detail, but one can picture no further. With the arch of the aorta unrolled, not only do the lungs become elongated, as they do when the spine is straightened, but now the spine seems to be "replicating" itself. Picturing the lungs spread out into one continuous sheet of gas exchange membrane is a more difficult task than imagining the surface of the small intestine straightened to the extent of a football field; it is both impossible and useless to imagine all these happening at the same time. But the aim here is not to visualize, but to quantify. What one will end up comparing is not the measures of different organs, regions, etc., but their respective metrics.

In light of the consequences of relativity, we can think of an absolute anatomy as Bólyaï's science of absolute space; in this view, studying the brain by considering its sections parallel to three planes will appear arbitrary, at best dictated by dire technical limitations. It is a different question whether this approach or any other will yield a better understanding of the intimate *function* of the brain, let alone the mind, but the benefits for clinical medicine and neurosurgery are quite easy to adumbrate.

From a broader scientific perspective, one ought to consider a different question. Classical mechanics is being taught and used for most of our practical needs, with no evident hindrance, and land surveyors are still plying their useful trade based on Ptolemaic astronomy; Sherlock Holmes also contended that for all he is concerned, the earth might as well revolve around the moon. But for those who—according, yet again, to Einstein (the author, this time, of the most unsettling pages of philosophy of science)[7]—will find favor with the angel of the Lord in charge of scientists, it will be necessary to articulate all the consequences of relativity for all branches of physics. Workers in other fields of science will be compelled to rethink their respective turfs, too. It is difficult to predict these consequences, but it is unlikely that our worldview will come out unscathed.

Admittedly, this is a tentative and general outline of a new approach to anatomy. It is, if not justified, at least with precedent, in G. F. Fitzgerald's modest contribution to the special theory of relativity. Two years after the Michelson-Morley experiment, Fitzgerald published a letter to the editor of *Science* magazine in which he proposed what is now remembered as the Fitzgerald contraction to explain the negative results of the crucial experiment. He did not live to see Hendrik Lorentz work out the more operational formula, much less the special theory of relativity, published sixteen years after Fitzgerald's communication. Aware of the strangeness of his brief note, Fitzgerald wrote his friend Oliver Heaviside on February 4, 1889: "*I admire from a distance those who contain themselves till they worked to the bottom of their results but as I am not in the very least sensitive to having made mistakes I rush out with all sorts of crude notions in hope that they might set others thinking and lead to some advance.*"

Peter Ratiu
Cambridge, July 2005

7. Albert Einstein, "Principles of Research," Address delivered at the celebration of Max Planck's sixtieth birthday before the Physical Society in Berlin (1918), in *Ideas and Opinions*, pp. 224–227.

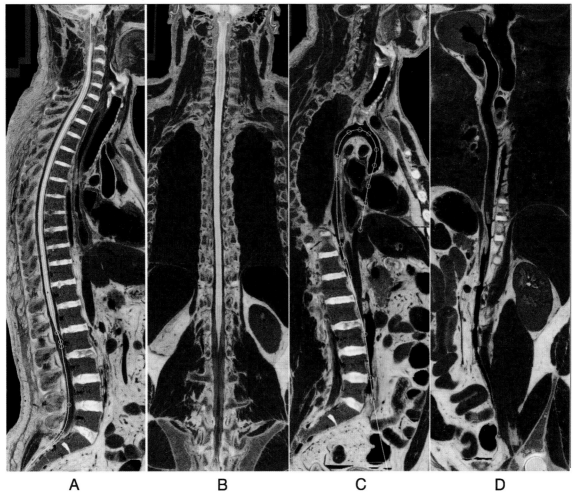

Figure 1. **A.** A slightly oblique parasagittal section, following the spinal cord. The trajectory of the curved surface along the spinal cord (**B**) is shown. **B.** The data block of the full specimen was sectioned about a surface passing through the spine and unrolled on a plane.
C. A slightly oblique parasagittal section. Parts of the aorta were caught in the section. The line indicates the direction of the entire aorta.
D. The data block was sectioned along the surface indicated in (**C**) and unrolled on a plane. The software employed did not permit two curvatures to be specified, which is why the arch of the aorta is not straight. (Illustrations derived from the Visible Human Male data set of the National Library of Medicine, using the Visible Human Server provided by the Ecole Polytechnique Fédérale de Lausanne, accessed at http://visiblehuman.epfl.ch.)

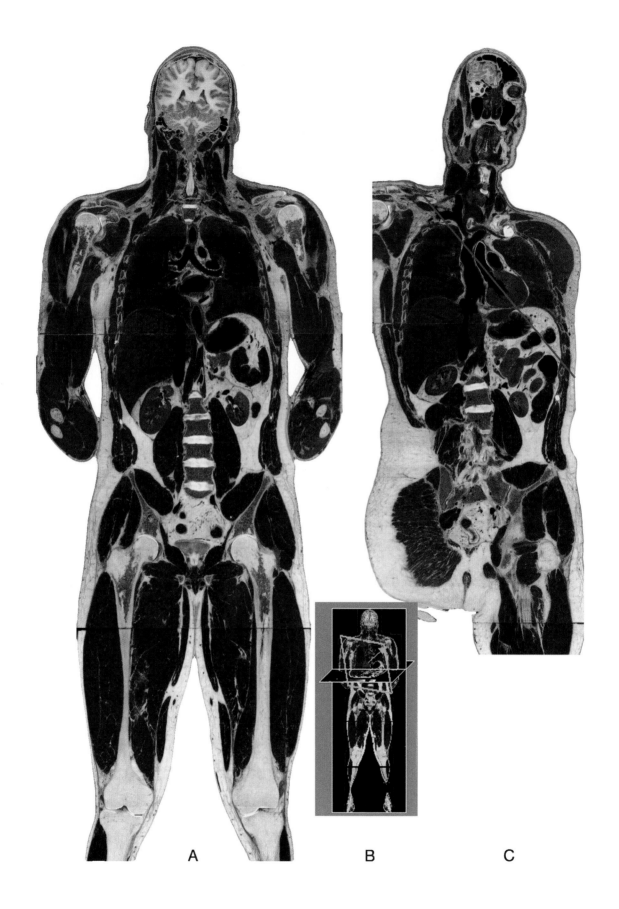

A

B

C

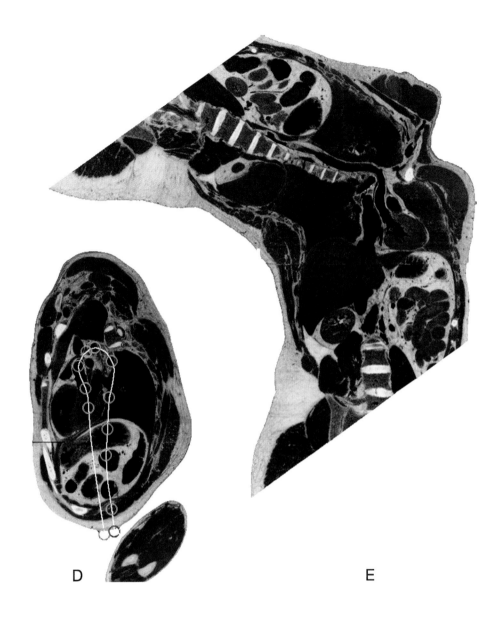

D   E

Figure 2. **A.** Coronal section through the body at the level of the posterior mediastinum. **B.** The green parallelogram indicates the angle of sectioning of the whole data block shown in (**C**). **C.** Oblique section through the body chosen to pass through the emergence of the aorta from the left ventricle. The blue line indicates the direction of the section in (**D**). **D.** Oblique section through the thorax. The line indicates the trajectory of a curved surface passing through the heart, ascending and descending aorta. **E.** The surface obtained along the line marked in (**D**), unrolled onto a plane. (Illustrations derived from the Visible Human Male data set of the National Library of Medicine, using the Visible Human Server provided by the Ecole Polytechnique Fédérale de Lausanne, accessed at http://visiblehuman.epfl.ch.)

Index

upper *ax1080, sag333, sag365, sag393, sag410, sag425, sag445, sag470, sag485, sag522*

Lobule

central—see cerebellum

inferior parietal *ax277, ax291, ax327, ax347, ax427, cor1140, cor1200, sag260, sag333*

paracentral *ax158, ax187, ax230, ax244, ax260, ax277, ax291, ax327, ax347, cor900, cor920, cor960, cor1000, cor1080, sag445, sag485, sag522*

superior parietal *ax230, ax244, ax260, ax277, ax291, ax327, ax347, ax367, ax382, ax410, ax427, cor1140, cor1200, sag260, sag290, sag333, sag365, sag393, sag410, sag425, sag445, sag470, sag485*

Long insular gyrus—see gyrus, insular

M

Mamillary body(-ies)—see body(-ies), mamillary

Mamillo-thalamic tract—see tract, mamillo-thalamic

Mandible *ax970, ax1045, ax1206, cor228, cor280, cor300, cor530, cor610, cor645, sag160, sag175, sag200, sag230, sag260, sag290, sag333, sag365, sag393, sag410, sag425, sag470, sag522*

head *ax899, ax926, ax944, cor450, cor712, cor721, cor744, cor760, sag75, sag110, sag130*

coronoid process *ax899, sag130*

ramus *ax1009, ax1080, cor570, cor675, cor712, cor721, sag110*

body *cor256, cor350, cor400, cor450, sag445*

Mandibular

fossa—see fossa

notch—*sag110*

Mastoid

cells *cor900, sag110, sag130, sag160*

process *ax858, ax899, ax926, ax944, ax970, ax1009, ax1080, cor818, cor860, cor900, cor920, cor1000, sag75, sag110, sag130, sag160, sag175*

Maxilla *sag260, sag290, sag333*

alveolar process *ax1080*

body *cor256, cor280, cor450*

zygomatic process *cor300, sag230*

Maxillary sinus—see sinus, paranasal maxillary

Meatus

acoustic

internal *ax830, cor818, cor860, sag260*

Medulla oblongata *ax830, ax899, ax926, ax944, ax970, ax1009, ax1045, cor860, cor920, cor960, cor1000, sag470, sag485, sag522*

Medullar

lamina *ax521, ax545*

velum

inferior *sag522*

superior *cor960, sag522*

Midbrain *sag425, sag470*

Muscle(-s)

buccinator *ax1045, ax1206, cor228, cor256, cor280, cor300, cor350, cor400, cor450, sag260*

depressor anguli oris *cor228, cor280, cor300*

digastric

anterior belly *cor256, cor280, cor300, cor350, cor400, cor450, cor818, sag333, sag365*

posterior belly *ax1080, cor860, cor900, cor1080, sag175, sag200, sag230, sag260*

epicranius—see muscle, occipitofrontalis

genioglossus *cor228, cor256, cor280, cor300, cor350, cor400, cor450, cor530, cor570, sag445, sag470, sag485, sag522*

geniohyoid *cor300, cor350, cor400, cor450, sag393, sag410, sag425, sag445, sag470, sag485, sag522*

hyoglossus *cor280, cor530, cor570*

inferior longitudinal (of the tongue) *cor400, cor530, cor570*

inferior rectus *ax780, cor280, cor300, cor350, cor400, cor450, sag260, sag290, sag333, sag365*

lateral pterygoid *ax899, ax926, ax944, ax970, cor450, cor530, cor645, cor721, sag160, sag290*

lower head *cor570, cor610, cor675, sag130, sag175, sag200, sag230, sag260*

upper head *cor570, cor610, cor675, sag175, sag200, sag230, sag260*

lateral rectus *ax711, ax747, cor280, cor300, cor350, cor400, cor450, sag290*

levator anguli oris *cor228*

levator labii superioris *cor228*

levator palpabrae superioris *cor300, cor400, cor450*

levator veli palatini *cor675, cor712, cor721, cor744, sag333, sag365*

longus capitis *ax944, ax970, ax1099, ax1045, ax1080, ax1206, cor744, cor760, cor920, sag333, sag365, sag393, sag410, sag425, sag445, sag470, sag485, sag522*

longus colli *cor860, sag333, sag393, sag410, sag425, sag445*

masseter *ax858, ax899, ax1009, ax1045, ax1206, cor450, cor530, cor570, cor610, cor645, cor675, sag75, sag110, sag130, sag160, sag175, sag200*

medial pterygoid *ax926, ax944, ax970, ax1009, ax1045, ax1080, ax1206, cor530, cor570, cor610, cor645, cor675, sag200, sag230, sag260, sag290, sag333*

medial rectus *ax660, ax691, ax711, ax747, cor256, cor280, cor300, cor350, cor400, cor450*

multifidus *sag230, sag260, sag290*

ax650, ax660, ax691, ax711, ax747, ax780, cor1080,
   cor1140, cor1200, sag522
      superior sagittal ax86, ax127, ax145, ax158, ax175,
         ax187, ax207, ax230, ax244, ax260, ax277, ax291,
         ax327, ax347, ax367, ax382, ax410, ax427, ax440,
         ax465, ax484, ax498, ax521, ax545, ax580, ax600,
         ax620, ax630, ax650, ax660, ax691, ax711, ax747,
         ax780, cor256, cor280, cor300, cor350, cor400,
         cor450, cor530, cor570, cor645, cor675, cor712, cor721,
         cor744, cor760, cor818, cor860, cor900, cor920,
         cor960, cor1000, cor1080, cor1140, cor1200, cor1275,
         cor1350, cor1377, sag470, sag522
      transverse ax780, ax830, cor1275, cor1350, sag230,
         sag260, sag290, sag333, sag365, sag393, sag410,
         sag425, sag445
Soft palate—see palate, soft
Spinal
   canal—see canal, spinal
   cord ax1206, cor1080, sag470, sag485, sag522
   nerve
      C2—sag410, sag425
      C3—sag425
Spinalis muscle—see muscle(-s), spinalis
Splenius capitis muscle—see muscle(-s), splenius capitis
Sternocleidomastoid muscle—see muscle(-s),
      sternocleidomastoid
Sternohyoid muscle—see muscle(-s), sternohyoid
Stria Genari—see area striata
Striatal gray matter bridges ax465
Striate area—see area striata
Subarachnoid space cor256
Subiculum—see hippocampus
Sublingual gland—see gland, sublingual
Submandibular gland, submandibular
Subparietal sulcus—see sulcus(-i), subparietal
Substantia
   nigra ax650, ax660, ax691 and ax691 closeup, cor744,
      cor760, cor818, sag425, sag445, sag470, sag485
   perforata anterior ax630, cor675
Subthalamic nucleus—see nucleus(-i), subthalamic
Sulcus(-i)
   calcarine ax521, ax545, ax580, ax600, ax620, cor960,
      cor1000, cor1080, cor1140, cor1200, cor1275, sag333,
      sag365, sag393, sag410, sag425, sag445, sag470, sag485
   central ax143, ax158, ax175, ax187, ax207, ax230, ax244,
      ax260, ax277, ax291, ax327, ax347, ax367, ax382,
      ax410, ax427, ax440, ax465, ax484, cor744, cor760,
      cor818, cor860, cor900, cor920, cor960, cor1000,
      sag110, sag130, sag160, sag175, sag200, sag230,

sag260, sag290, sag333, sag365, sag393, sag410,
   sag425, sag445, sag470
cingulate ax521, ax545, ax580, cor450, cor610, cor645,
   cor675, cor712, cor721, cor744, cor760, cor810,
   cor860, cor900, cor960, cor1080, sag445, sag470,
   sag522
collateral ax630, ax650, ax660, ax691, ax711, ax747,
   cor645, cor675, cor712, cor920, cor960, cor1000,
   cor1080, cor1140, sag260, sag333, sag365
inferior frontal ax367, ax382, cor350, cor400, cor450,
   cor530, cor570, cor645
inferior temporal cor610, cor645, cor675, cor712, cor744,
   cor760, cor860, cor900, cor920, cor960, cor1000,
   cor1080, cor1140, sag200
insular
   central cor570, cor712
   circular cor570, cor645, cor675, cor712, cor721, cor744
intraparietal ax382, ax410, ax427, ax440, cor1140, cor1200,
   sag260, sag333
lateral (Sylvius) ax545, ax580, ax600, ax620, ax630,
   ax650, ax660, ax691, cor530, cor570, cor610, cor645,
   cor675, cor712, cor721, cor744, cor760, cor860,
   cor900, cor920, cor960, cor1000, cor1080, sag110,
   sag130, sag160, sag175, sag200, sag230, sag260,
   sag290, sag333
occipitotemporal cor744, cor760, cor818, cor860, cor900,
   cor960, cor1000, cor1080, cor1140
olfactory ax620, ax630, ax650, cor400, cor450, cor530,
   cor570, sag445
parietooccipital ax465, ax498, cor1080, cor1140, cor1200,
   cor1275, sag230, sag260, sag290, sag445
postcentral ax230, ax244, ax260, ax277, ax291, ax327,
   ax347, ax367, ax382, cor860, cor900, cor920,
   cor960, cor1000, cor1080, sag175, sag260, sag290,
   sag333, sag365, sag410, sag425, sag470, sag485
precentral ax127, ax143, sag175, ax187, ax207, ax230,
   ax277, ax291, ax367, ax382, ax410, ax440, cor675,
   cor712, cor721, cor744, cor760, cor818, cor860,
   sag290, sag333, sag365, sag393, sag410, sag425
rhinal cor645, cor675, cor712, cor744, cor760, cor818,
   cor860, cor900, cor920
subparietal cor1000, sag445
superior frontal ax143, ax158, ax175, ax187, ax207, ax230,
   ax244, ax260, ax277, ax291, ax327, ax347, ax367,
   ax382, cor280, cor300, cor350, cor400, cor450, cor530,
   cor570, cor610, cor645, cor675, cor712, cor721, cor744,
   cor760, cor818, cor960, sag260, sag333, sag365,
   sag445
superior temporal cor570, cor675, cor712, cor744, cor760,

cor818, cor860, cor900, cor920, cor1000, cor1080, cor1140, sag27, sag45, sag75, sag110, sag130, sag160, sag175, sag200

Supramarginal gyrus—see gyrus, supramarginal

Supraoptic recess—see third ventricle

Suprapineal recess—see third ventricle

Suture

    lambdoid sag75, sag110, sag130, sag160, sag175, sag230

T

Tarsus

    lower ax780, sag290

    upper ax711, ax747

Temporal

    gyrus(-i)

        inferior—see gyrus, temporal

        middle—see gyrus, temporal

        superior—see gyrus, temporal

        transverse (Heschl)—see gyrus, temporal

    sulcus(-i)

        superior—see sulcus, temporal superior

        inferior—see sulcus, temporal inferior

Temporalis

    fascia ax382, ax410, ax427, ax440, ax498, ax521, ax600, ax620, ax630, ax650, ax747, ax830, cor530, cor570, cor610, cor645, cor712, cor721, cor744

    muscle—see muscle(-s), temporalis

Temporo-mandibular

    articular disc cor712, cor721, cor744, cor760, sag75, sag110, sag130, sag160

    joint ax858, ax899, cor712, cor721, cor744, cor760, sag75, sag110, sag130, sag160

Tentorium cerebelli ax600, ax620, ax630, ax650, ax660, ax691, ax711, ax747, cor721, cor744, cor760, cor818, cor860, cor900, cor920, cor960, cor1000, cor1080, cor1140, cor1200, cor1275, sag160, sag175, sag200, sag230, sag260, sag333, sag365, sag393 and sag393 closeup, sag410, sag425, sag445, sag470, sag485

Thalamostriate vein—see vein(-s), thalamostriate

Thalamus

    nucleus(-i)—see nucleus(-i), thalamic

Third ventricle—see ventricle, third

Thyreoglossal duct cor610, cor645, cor675, sag445, sag470, sag485, sag522

Thyrohyoid

    membrane cor675, sag365, sag393, sag410, sag425

    muscle—see muscle(-s), thyrohyoid

Thyroid cartilage—see cartilage, thyroid

Tongue

    body ax1206, cor280, cor300, cor350, cor450, cor610, cor645, cor675, sag333, sag365, sag393, sag410, sag425, sag470, sag485

    mucosa cor400, cor530, cor570, sag445, sag522

    muscle

        inferior longitudinal—see muscle(-s), inferior longitudinal of tongue

        superior longitudinal—see muscle(-s), superior longitudinal of tongue

        transverse—see muscle(-s), transverse of tongue

        vertical—see muscle(-s), vertical of tongue

Tooth(-eeth)

    canine

        left inferior ax1206, cor228

        right inferior sag425

    incisor

        left central inferior ax1206

        left lateral inferior ax1206, cor228

    premolar 1, left inferior cor228

Tract

    mamillo-thalamic ax600, ax620, ax630, cor721, cor744, cor760

    olfactory ax691, cor400, cor450

    optic ax650, ax660, cor675, cor712, cor721, cor744, sag393 and sag393 closeup, sag410, sag425, sag445, sag470, sag522

Transverse

    ligament of atlas—see ligament, transverse of atlas

    sinus—see sinus, venous transverse

    temporal gyri (Heschl)—see gyrus, temporal

Trigeminal

    ganglion (Gasser) ax780

    nerve (CN V)—see nerve(-s), trigeminal

Trochlear nerve (CN IV)—see nerve(-s), trochlear

U

Uncal vein—see vein(-s), uncal

Uncinate gyrus—see gyrus(-i), uncinate

Uvula

    of cerebellum—see cerebellum

    soft palate cor712, cor721, sag485

V

Valecula sag425, sag470, sag485, sag522

Ventral

    anterior nucleus of thalamus—see nucleus(-i), anterior thalamic